Complementary medicine and disability

Alternatives for people with disabling conditions

Andrew Vickers

Research Council for Complementary Medicine
London, UK

CHAPMAN & HALL

London · Glasgow · New York · Tokyo · Melbourne · Madras

Published by Chapman & Hall, 2–6 Boundary Row, London SE1 8HN

Chapman & Hall, 2–6 Boundary Row, London SE1 8HN, UK

Blackie Academic & Professional, Wester Cleddens Road, Bishopbriggs, Glasgow G64 2NZ, UK

Chapman & Hall Inc., One Penn Plaza, 41st Floor, New York NY10119, USA

Chapman & Hall Japan, Thomson Publishing Japan, Hirakawacho Nemoto Building, 6F, 1–7–11 Hirakawa-cho, Chiyoda-ku, Tokyo 102, Japan

Chapman & Hall Australia, Thomas Nelson Australia, 102 Dodds Street, South Melbourne, Victoria 3205, Australia

Chapman & Hall India, R. Seshadri, 32 Second Main Road, CIT East, Madras 600 035, India

Distributed in the USA and Canada by Singular Publishing Group Inc., 4284 41st Street, San Diego, California 92105

First edition 1993

© 1993 Andrew Vickers

Typeset in 10/12 Palatino by Mews Photosetting, Beckenham, Kent
Printed in Great Britain by St Edmundsbury Press, Bury St Edmunds, Suffolk

ISBN 0 412 48690 3   1 56593 232 3 (USA)

A catalogue record for this book is available from the British Library

Library of Congress Cataloging-in-Publication data available

∞ Printed on permanent acid-free text paper, manufactured in accordance with ANSI/NISO Z 39.48–1992 and ANSI Z 39.48–1984

Contents

Contents

Part IV Appendices

Preface

This book aims to allow people with physical disabilities to make informed decisions about complementary medicine. I have written it because I believe that individuals should take control and personal responsibility for their healthcare, especially where health problems are long-term or serious. For this to occur, it is essential that suitable and accurate information is available. However, much writing and information about complementary medicine is largely inappropriate to the needs of people with disabilities: few books discuss health problems which are common amongst disabled people or see disability as an important context for healthcare. The doctrine of 'perfect health' espoused by many texts (often accompanied by images of the young and able-bodied) similarly ignores the dimension of disability.

Moreover, few books or leaflets about complementary medicine are authored by independent observers. Most are written by those who have a vested interest in 'selling' a particular story to the reader: the typical author is a practitioner of orthodox or complementary medicine who is often more interested in stating his or her personal views about medicine than in allowing readers to come to practical decisions of their own. The giving of independent advice so that individuals can make practical decisions is the prime aim of this book.

Sickness, health and disability

One of the difficulties in writing this book has been that, in discussing health, it has been necessary to discuss health problems. This might give the impression that disabled people are sick and weak; that they should receive medical attention (gratefully) from the able-bodied; that the barriers which disabled people face are located within their own bodies, rather than in society; in general, that being disabled is something to be 'endured' or 'suffered'. I can only say that these are not opinions I hold. I would like to take this opportunity to state that:

- I wholeheartedly endorse the campaigns to make disability an issue of rights, rather than charity.
- I fully support legislation on access, transport and employment which seeks to sanction unfair discrimination against disabled people.
- I am committed to the use of positive language which stresses that people with disabilities are individuals.
- I am against the use of words and images which encourage or provoke pity and dependence.
- I accept that healthcare is not, and should not be, the prime concern of people with disabilities.

Explanations of some terms

I take 'disability' as referring to conditions which cause long-term and substantial difficulties in leading a normal life. There is no hard and fast distinction between able-bodiedness and disability and I accept that there are many 'grey areas'. One of the 'grey areas' I have included is that of people who are not disabled but who have potentially disabling conditions such as multiple sclerosis. On the other hand, it has been necessary to restrict mention of some categories of disability: common health problems in asthma or epilepsy, for example, show only marginal similarities to those found in physical disabilities such as rheumatoid arthritis, cerebral palsy or stroke and therefore are not covered in great detail.

There may also be some confusion over the use of the term 'healthcare'; after all, disabled people are not 'ill'. I would like to make a distinction, however, between being ill and having a health problem. Many people, able-bodied and disabled alike, have problems with their health, even though they may not be technically 'ill'. The health problems I discuss in this book are those which disabled people have reported to have been helped by complementary medicine. Some, such as irritable bowel syndrome, insomnia or just a general lack of vitality, are also common in the able-bodied; others, such as spasm or impaired sensation, are more particular to disability. It is also worth pointing out that many people try complementary medicine not because they have a specific health problem as such, but because they are interested in achieving a greater level of general well-being.

Finally ... this book is intended to be informative, not definitive. There are inherent methodological problems in writing and researching a book for a lay audience and these have precluded any firm and eternal conclusions. It has not been my intention to put before you the one and only truth about complementary medicine and disability: I aim merely to present a general guide to help you come to your own decisions about health and healthcare.

The names and several other details of many of the individuals mentioned in this book have been changed so as to ensure confidentiality.

Acknowledgements

This book is dedicated to my mother, who pointed out the pianists' posture.

Far more people have helped with this project than can be listed here: to all of those who have shared personal experiences, or who have offered help and advice, many thanks. Special mention must go to:

Gill Levy; Jane Foulkes of the Institute for Complementary Medicine; Holly Gothard – my editor; Peter Davies of the Marylebone Centre Trust for help with bibliographic searches; Steve Vogel; Sue Cartlidge; Andrew Bates; Dr Martin Allbright; Nora Franglen; Maria North; Sally Martin; Marilyn Bear; Batya Parker; Shirley Brookner; Gaston St Pierre; the SCOPE practitioners: Suzanne Adamson, Hilary Leacock, Christine Mathieson, Nicholas Pole; the staff and users of Warwick Row; Robin Monro of the Yoga Biomedical Trust; Julia Segal of ARMS; Islington Crossroads; Linda Broda; Ann Lett of the British School of Reflex Zone Therapy of the Feet; Dr Peter Fisher of the Royal London Homoeopathic Hospital; Dr June Burger; Sarah Williams of the Council for Acupuncture; Dr J Brostoff; JP Scott; Caroline Kettle of the Hoxton Health Group; Helen Sanderson; Ann Warren Davies; Liz Scannel; Deborah Cackler; Tom Harding for computer advice; Jack and Lily Levy, Jo and Angela Vickers, Terry and Steve Berzon for help with the computer; Saul Berkovitz for many discussions; Cath Chadwick for many things; Jeff Vickers.

Funding acknowledgements are due to Sir Charles Jessel's Charitable Trust and the Research Council for Complementary Medicine.

Acknowledgements

Photographic acknowledgements photographs/illustrations provided by: Leon Morris; National Institute of Medical Herbalists; Osteopathic Information Service; John Smith and The Register of Traditional Chinese Medicine. The remaining photographs were taken by the author. Thanks are due to: Steve Berzon; Natural Remedies and Bumblebees; Sarah Laing and PALACE; Florence Crabtree and the users of Highbury New Park; The Centre for Training; Hedwig Verdonk.

Permissions acknowledgements Faber & Faber for permission to quote from *Multiple sclerosis: exploring sickness and health* by Elizabeth Forsythe. The Evening Standard for permission to quote Dr Peter May. The Houghton Mifflin Company for permission to quote from *Health and healing* Copyright © 1983 by Andrew Weil (all rights reserved). Random Century Group, Arcadia and Harper Collins Publishers for permission to quote from *Peace, love and healing* by Bernie Siegel.

Part one

Complementary healthcare: an introduction and overview

1

Introduction to complementary medicine

WHAT IS COMPLEMENTARY MEDICINE?

Techniques such as acupuncture, homoeopathy, massage and yoga are generally described as 'complementary' medicine. This seems to suggest that the different therapies somehow form a single body of knowledge. In fact, each has developed as a separate tradition along independent lines.

- Acupuncture originated in China many thousands of years ago and is based upon traditional Oriental views about health.
- Homoeopathy was founded in Europe in the late 18th century and is now used by orthodox physicians in many parts of the world.
- Massage has been used in almost all cultures throughout history.
- Yoga was first practised in India in ancient times.

There are many other complementary therapies, each of which has its own particular techniques and traditions (see the box on pages 6–8). It is not easy to explain why, despite so much variation, these different therapies have been given the single label 'complementary medicine'.

Some people say that complementary medicine can be defined as that which involves ideas about the body or health or treatment which are not found in conventional medicine. In this view, what makes a therapy 'complementary' is only that it is not yet conventional. Patrick Pietroni, a London GP who is prominently involved in complementary medicine, says that talking about complementary therapies is a bit like talking about foreigners: we can't say what they are, only what they are not.

However, many complementary therapies do share a number of common characteristics. Perhaps one of the most basic is the belief that the body has an inherent ability to heal itself and that the aim of treatment should be to stimulate and enhance this capacity. Take the case of recurrent colds and 'flu, a common problem in some disabled people. The orthodox approach is to prescribe a course of antibiotics to kill off the bacteria causing the infection. A homoeopath, on the other hand, might prescribe a remedy to strengthen the person's constitution, so that his or her body would better able to fight the infection for itself. An acupuncturist would attempt much the same feat by working with the energy which is believed to flow through the body.

Many people say that another characteristic which unites the complementary therapies is that their approach to health care is 'holistic'. Holistic is a tricky word, and it often comes to mean whatever a speaker wants it to mean. However, it is normally taken as referring to therapies which consider the physical, emotional, spiritual, mental, and social sides of an individual with respect to what causes ill-health, how it should be treated and what the aim of that treatment should be.

Holistic causes Traditionally, orthodox medicine tends to look for a specific cause of disease, for example, an infectious agent such as a virus. Holistic medicine involves the belief that what causes ill-health cannot be reduced to such a single cause: many aspects of individuals and their environment contribute to causing the state in which they become susceptible to ill-health.

Holistic treatment Orthodox medicine generally treats only the physical body: surgery to remove a cancerous growth is a good example of this. A holistic practitioner would also be interested in an individual's mind, emotions and physical and social environment.

Holistic aims Sometimes, orthodox practitioners will consider their work done once the physical body is 'fixed'. In holistic forms of medicine, the goal of physical improvement is complemented by the attempt to improve the mental, emotional and spiritual well-being of the individual. This difference, between aiming to remove or suppress the physical manifestations of disease and aiming to maximize the potential of the whole individual is sometimes described as the difference between 'curing' and 'healing'.

Some authorities have pointed out that many good orthodox doctors take a holistic approach. So, if holism is indeed a characteristic of complementary medicine, it is not a unique one. A similar point can be made about the relationship between practitioner and client in complementary medicine. Talking and discussion, often of a personal nature, are seen by many as important aspects of complementary treatment and so the degree of trust, empathy and respect between practitioner and client is taken to be vital to its outcome. Though the relationship that many people have with their complementary practitioner is markedly different to that which they have with their orthodox doctor, many physicians do build up good, equal relationships with their patients.

One feature which does seem to distinguish complementary medicine, is that treatment is generally gentle and pleasant: technological and invasive procedures are avoided and negative side-effects are rare. One upshot of this is that people who have no particular health problems at all often visit complementary practitioners. Techniques such as massage, shiatsu and tai chi are wonderfully relaxing and enjoyable and can be used for the pure pleasure they bring.

An associated issue is that, whereas in orthodox medicine the 'patient' tends to play an entirely passive role as the recipient of therapy, the user of complementary medicine is generally an active participant in treatment. This participation not only includes dietary change, and the practice of techniques such as meditation, yoga or movement exercise, it also extends to taking personal responsibility for healthcare and to making decisions about how treatment should proceed.

Finally, one of the most interesting, and controversial, aspects of the complementary therapies is that they often involve ideas which diverge from conventional scientific understanding. For example, reflexologists say that the organs and structures of the body are represented on the feet: needless to say, this is not shared by many anatomists. It remains to be explained why therapies which seem to conflict with science also seem to work.

DIFFERENT TYPES OF COMPLEMENTARY MEDICINE

There are many different forms of complementary medicine. A brief summary of each is given in the box below. It is clear that some of the therapies and techniques listed, for example, yoga or counselling, are difficult to class as 'medicine' even though they may help resolve 'medical' problems. This is why the term 'complementary healthcare' is used for much of this book.

A brief introduction to the complementary therapies

A number of short descriptions are given below to help you through the first four chapters of the book: more information on each therapy can be found in Chapter 5.

Massage
Massage is technically described as the 'manipulation of soft tissue'. Massage in complementary healthcare tends towards the more gentle and comforting, rather than the harsh and vigorous.

Aromatherapy
Some practitioners use essential oils distilled from plants when they give massage. These are believed to have benefits such as increasing blood circulation or breaking down mucus. Aromatherapy oils can also be used in compresses, baths and vaporizers.

Reflexology
This is a type of foot massage in which certain areas of the foot are believed to correspond to areas of the body: stimulation of the foot is believed to bring about healing in other parts of the body.

Healing
More widely known as spiritual healing, or the laying on of hands, this therapy does not, in fact, require a religious context. For example, some nurses in the US practice a form of healing as part of their daily hospital work.

The metamorphic technique/polarity
Perhaps best thought of as a special type of healing (see previous paragraph).

Acupuncture
This is the well known technique of inserting needles into the skin at special points. The basis of acupuncture is that health is determined by the flow of internal energy through the body and that needles can be used to correct imbalances in this flow.

Shiatsu
This is a form of Japanese massage which uses pressure on special points on the body. It can be seen as a halfway house between massage and acupuncture.

Osteopathy and chiropractic
By massaging muscle and soft tissue in a special way, and by manipulating joints (popularly thought of as 'cracking bones'), practitioners of osteopathy and chiropractic can relieve pain and stiffness and improve mobility.

Rolfing
Originating in America, this technique uses strong pressure to reorganize the structures of the body.

Alexander technique
This is a way of learning how to use the body efficiently in everyday life. Alexander teachers say that good use of the body can improve mobility and help with pain problems.

Feldenkrais
In some ways simlar to Alexander, Feldenkrais uses gentle exercises and a technique somewhat akin to a light massage.

Relaxation, meditation and creative visualization
These are self-help techniques which are normally learnt at a class and practised every day at home. As well as promoting general well-being, the techniques can be used for specific therapeutic purposes.

Yoga
This combines meditation and breathing exercises with special postures which are thought to improve the functioning of the body. Yoga is a self-help technique which can be practised at home.

Tai chi
A gentle movement exercise which originates from China. The most well-known part of tai chi is the 'solo form': a series of slow and graceful movements which follow a set pattern.

Homoeopathy
This therapy uses very small doses of common substances in pill form. In some ways similar to orthodox medicine (the prescription of tablets), homoeopathy is actually based on very different principles.

Herbal medicine
Most simply thought of as the use of herbs to remedy disease, though different herbalists may prescribe in different ways.

Nutrition
Changing the diet can have important effects on health. Some nutritionists also prescribe vitamin and mineral supplements.

Naturopathy
Practitioners of naturopathy combine nutritional therapy, osteopathy and herbal medicine.

Counselling
Talking things through with a counsellor can help people to cope with and overcome emotional difficulties and distress.

Hypnotherapy
More of a self-help technique than 'falling under another's power', hypnotherapy can be an effective technique for relaxation and for allaying some symptoms.

COMPLEMENTARY HEALTHCARE DOES NOT REPLACE
ORTHODOX MEDICINE

Many of the therapies mentioned in this book are called 'alternative medicine' by some people. This seems to suggest that they are something you might consider doing instead of seeing your doctor. The term 'complementary' is now favoured by many workers because it suggests that it is, of course, possible to do both: going for a massage, taking up yoga or using homoeopathic remedies are all things which can be done in addition to any treatment suggested by an orthodox physician.

There are a number of different ways of thinking about the relationship between orthodox and complementary medicine. Some physicians put forward a kind of 'division of labour' argument in which orthodox medicine takes care of the physical body and complementary practitioners are left to look after our psychological and social sides. Others see the role of complementary healthcare as primarily preventative: massage, meditation, yoga and the like are seen to reduce levels of stress and this can help prevent a number of health problems, for example, high blood pressure.

However, neither of these points of view reflects what happens in complementary healthcare in practice. Complementary healthcare can in fact be seen as preventative, though in a more specific sense, reducing the number of attacks of a disease, but leaving the treatment of the attacks which do occur to orthodox measures. For example, people with asthma who practise yoga often experience fewer attacks of breathlessness, though once an attack has actually started, they will normally resort to using an aerosol puffer to dilate the airways. In a similar way, some people who have visited acupuncturists for the treatment of arthritis still use drugs when they get severe bouts of pain, though many say that this occurs less frequently since starting treatment.

Complementary and conventional medicine may also work directly side by side: acupuncture, for example, may be found alongside more conventional treatments in the pain clinics of many hospitals; in one study of homoeopathy, patients who were given both orthodox drugs and homoeopathy were found to do better than those who took orthodox drugs alone.

In rehabilitation work, complementary and orthodox treatments can work hand in hand, each addressing those problems to which it is most suited. For example, osteopathy might help muscle pain following a hip replacement operation. As another example, a physiotherapist and an Alexander teacher might co-operate in various ways: the physiotherapist might first build up a patient's strength so that an Alexander teacher could help her to move more efficiently. Alternatively, an Alexander teacher might work on an individual's awareness of his body so that he could do his physiotherapy exercises more effectively.

By combining complementary and orthodox medicine in certain ways, some individuals have managed to get the best of both worlds, utilizing what each has to offer in order to get the maximum benefit.

In Chapter 4, you can find a discussion of how to decide on a programme of healthcare to overcome health problems and maximize general well-being. What appears to be true is that in the majority of cases, the best programmes involve elements of both complementary and orthodox medicine. The two forms of medicine are not competing 'alternatives'. Each offers a set of resources which individuals can employ to best effect. This is why complementary healthcare should not be seen to replace orthodox medicine.

HOW COMPLEMENTARY HEALTHCARE IS PRACTISED

Many practitioners of complementary medicine do not have orthodox medical qualifications. Typically a practitioner will have undergone a two or three year training at a special school and become registered with a suitable professional organization after qualifying. The practitioner will then start up a practice, often converting a room in his or her own home for this purpose.

Generally speaking, complementary medicine is private medicine. The schools and registering bodies do not receive state support and must survive on the fees they are able to generate. Moreover, unlike those working on the NHS, practitioners must be paid directly by their clients for the services they provide.

Practitioners of complementary healthcare are not subject to the same laws and regulations as their orthodox counterparts: for example, whereas only those registered with the General Medicine Council may call themselves medical doctors, anyone at all, regardless of skills and training, can set themselves up as an acupuncturist or homoeopath.

There is no single governing body for all practitioners of complementary healthcare; in fact, there are often several governing bodies for a single therapy. Practitioners can train in a number of different schools and these schools vary in the length and intensity of the course offered, the approach of the teaching and the method of qualifying. In addition, certain complementary techniques have sub-disciplines and competing styles. As a result, practitioners doing essentially the same kind of work may have different qualifications and be registered by different organizations.

This leads to the great problem of complementary healthcare, which is that the competence of those who practise it varies widely. On the one hand, there are orthodox doctors with 30 years experience of using complementary techniques; on the other, there are those without a previous interest or qualification in medicine who become practitioners after a weekend reflexology course. This is one of the reasons why individuals seeking complementary health services must use care and discretion in their choice of therapy and practitioner. Suitable advice on this matter can be found in Chapter 4.

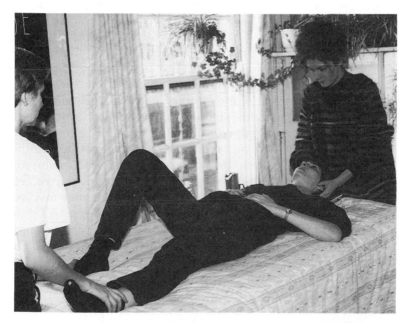

Figure 1.1 Students learning the Alexander technique. Broadly speaking, there is no public funding of complementary healthcare: the majority of practitioners have no orthodox medical qualifications and train at private institutions.

The situation is changing however. Firstly, it is likely that chiropractic and osteopathy will be granted special legal status in the near future; moreover, an organization called the Institute for Complementary Medicine has been granted the right to set up a British Register of Complementary Practitioners. In league with a government agency, the National Council for Vocational Qualifications, the Institute has also been working to establish a national system of assessment and qualification. Though much of their work is to be applauded, the Institute for Complementary Medicine has not received backing from all groups in the world of complementary medicine and it is still a matter for conjecture whether the British Register will attain universal recognition or will remain just as one useful resource among many.

SELF-HELP OR PROFESSIONAL HELP?

Many people seem to think that complementary healthcare is primarily about self-help: in this view, the alternative to the doctor's surgery is the health store, with its bottles of herbal remedies and vitamin pills, and the bookshop, with its 'How To ... ' health and diet guides. The problem is, of course, that healthcare is more complicated than a book, or a bottle of pills, might suggest. For example, a health store might sell a herbal tablet for 'arthritis'. However, there are many different types of arthritis and each condition involves symptoms other than joint pain. Moreover, recovery from an arthritic condition may require physiotherapy to improve and maintain mobility. It is also worth pointing out that illness often involves psychological and personal issues and that healing may involve more than just looking at swollen joints.

Professional practitioners of medicine have experience and understanding of healthcare. They are also able to offer skilled techniques, such as osteopathy to ease an arthritic joint or acupuncture to help with pain. Finally, practitioners are able to offer their energy and support; after all, healing can be a long and difficult process and illness is both physically and emotionally draining.

So if an individual has a serious health problem, he or she should seriously consider involving a professional practitioner in the treatment. Though self-help has many advantages, and though it often plays an important role in complementary therapy, it should essentially be seen as an additional resource.

Seeking professional help, however, can bring its own problems. Professionals can sometimes act, or be treated by their clients, as 'experts' and they can sometimes take, or be given, power over other people's lives on the authority of their technical knowledge. Furthermore, the mere act of consulting a professional may decrease a person's sense of self-reliance and self-worth.

It is important that people who wish to use complementary healthcare are aware of these potential difficulties. Professionals are perhaps best seen as 'enablers', who help individuals to achieve their aims, rather than as experts. This suggests a more equal role for practitioner and client; in fact, some workers describe the ideal relationship as a 'therapeutic partnership' in which mutual trust, empathy and respect are the key elements.

Chapter 13 is exclusively dedicated to the subject of self-help; Chapter 14 contains further discussion on the role of individuals in healthcare and the relationship between client and practitioner.

DOES IT WORK?

The question of whether or not a complementary therapy 'works' is complicated – and highly contentious. Whereas some people contend that the experience of millions of people over many centuries is proof enough, others argue that subjective experience is entirely irrelevant and that only careful scientific study should be trusted. This section is concerned with this latter view and examines the scientific evidence on complementary healthcare.

Medical research on complementary healthcare is beset by a number of problems. One of the most intractable is how to control for the 'placebo effect'. This is when the mere suggestion that a therapy might be beneficial brings about an improvement (see page 55 for more about placebos). In trials of drugs, controlling for the placebo effect causes few problems: one group of patients receives the drug while another group is given a pill which contains no active medicine. Thinking up a placebo for acupuncture, osteopathy or massage is less easy. How do you give a fake massage?

Moreover, a requirement of most research trials is that they should be 'double blind'; in other words, neither the patients nor the practitioners should know who is receiving the real treatment. In most complementary therapies, it would be impossible for practitioners to remain unaware that they were giving a treatment.

There is the additional problem that most studies take the form 'Therapy A for Condition B' (e.g. acupuncture for chronic pain, aspirin for rheumatic pain). Complementary practitioners may give different diagnoses, and therefore different treatments, to individuals who have identical diseases, according to their orthodox doctors.

Despite all these problems, the medical literature provides us with considerable, if not indubitable, evidence that complementary healthcare can be a safe and effective form of treatment. It is simply not true that, as so often stated, 'complementary therapies have never been the subject of well-controlled studies printed in major medical journals'.

The following is a summary of the most important recent research. Appropriate references can be found in the bibliography.

Homoeopathy

In 1991, three Dutch researchers (Kleijnen, Knipschild and ter Riet) conducted an extensive review of published studies of homoeopathy. The authors state clearly that they were initially sceptical:

> We could not believe the positive result [of one trial] . . . and therefore started to search for further reports.

The researchers located 107 papers, 81 of which gave a result which was favourable to homoeopathy. In the most scientifically rigorous trials, homoeopathy was successful 15 times out of 22. The researchers commented:

> The amount of positive evidence even among the best studies came as a surprise to us. Based on this evidence, we would be ready to accept that homoeopathy can be

efficacious, if only the mechanism of its action were more plausible.

In other words, if homoeopathy had been scientifically studied and understood, there would be little doubt of its effectiveness.

Acupuncture

There have been a surprisingly large number of scientific studies on acupuncture. It is partly because of these studies that acupuncture has become one of the more widely accepted complementary therapies: its use in orthodox pain clinics, for example, is now commonplace.

Studies of acupuncture for pain often show that though it has benefits, these are not statistically significant. This may result from the difficulties involved in acupuncture research or from the wide variation found in responses to acupuncture in a research situation, where some subjects appear to do very well and others appear to remain unaffected. In any event, because most studies do favour acupuncture, pooling the results (a statistical technique known as meta-analysis) does give a statistically significant positive result for acupuncture research as a whole. As one reviewer, Charles Vincent, put it, despite the confusions and complications of acupuncture research, the efficacy of acupuncture 'is greater than would be expected from a placebo'.

A number of major medical journals have published research concerned with the treatment, by acupuncture, of conditions other than pain. A typical paper studied 'disabling breathlessness'. After a course of treatment, subjects felt less breathless and could walk further in a set period of time, though laboratory tests of lung function showed no improvement. Again, individual variation was very high: on a 5-point score of shortness of breath, some subjects remained at 1 whereas others went up to 5 which indicated 'Being able to keep up with people of a similar age on the level'.

Despite many studies apparently favourable to acupuncture, some authorities have expressed doubt, pointing out that most trials have been of insufficient rigour.

Herbal medicine

A large number of modern medicines have been developed from herbal remedies. One of the best-known is aspirin, which is a chemically synthesized version of a compound found in the bark of willow trees. This is one of the reasons that few orthodox doctors have difficulties with the idea that herbal remedies can be effective, in some instances at least. Another reason is that there have been a number of positive clinical and laboratory trials of herbal formulations. For example, in one trial of a herbal remedy for osteoarthritis, levels of both pain and disability dropped significantly. In another trial, an extract of various root barks and nuts was shown to improve experimentally induced arthritis in rats. Other successful studies have shown the benefits of herbs for seasickness, insomnia, eczema and wound healing.

Nutrition

There is a widespread agreement that certain dietary changes, for example, reducing the intake of sugar and saturated fats, can play an important role in preventing a number of diseases. Moreover, a number of scientifically rigorous studies have demonstrated that dietary manipulation can be an effective treatment for specific conditions. Food intolerance diets (see the section on Nutrition in Chapter 11) have been shown to be of benefit in rheumatoid arthritis, irritable bowel syndrome and asthma. Modification of the fat content of the diet has shown to be of benefit in rheumatoid arthritis, multiple sclerosis and a number of other conditions.

The evidence on the use of vitamin and mineral supplements is less straightforward. Though some studies have demonstrated benefit (e.g. pantothenate and copper for rheumatoid arthritis) many studies seem to show no effect (e.g. zinc for rheumatoid arthritis). Perhaps the most appropriate conclusion is that, if used discerningly by well qualified individuals, vitamin and mineral supplementation might be beneficial in certain cases.

Manipulative medicine (chiropractic, osteopathy, Rolfing)

A study of chiropractic for low back pain was published in the *British Medical Journal* in 1990. The report concluded that:

> For patients with low back pain .... chiropractic almost certainly confers worthwhile, long-term benefit in comparison with hospital outpatient management. The benefit is seen most in those with chronic and severe pain. Introducing chiropractic into the NHS should be considered.

Although generally favourable, other studies, including those on osteopathy, have had more mixed results, partly as a result of the difficulties in designing adequate trials. A study of Rolfing for cerebral palsy indicated that it could be an effective treatment for 'mildly impaired patients'.

Alexander technique

Though the Alexander technique has not yet been subject to rigorous trial, a number of studies have demonstrated benefit. Findings have included: improved respiratory function in healthy volunteers after a course of Alexander training; that Alexander training was the most helpful technique in a pain management programme as rated by patients; that Alexander training led to improved posture and balance.

Hypnotherapy

Well-controlled trials of hypnotherapy have been conducted for various conditions, including asthma, pain and irritable bowel syndrome. Most results have been positive.

Therapies which involve relaxation

Studies of yoga, meditation and relaxation have demonstrated beneficial effects in a number of conditions including high blood pressure, pain and asthma. It is believed that all relaxation techniques result in a similar set of beneficial physical changes in the body. This is called the 'relaxation response' and is discussed in the section on meditation in Chapter 10

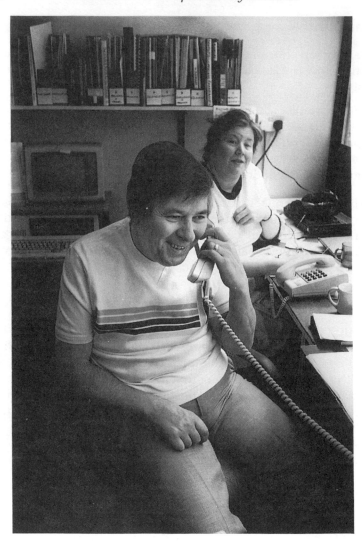

Figure 1.2 Bill Mann in the offices of the Westminster Disability Information Service. Bill has received reflexology for a number of years. He says that one of the biggest changes has been in his general sense of well-being: 'I feel "bubbly" now'.

(see page 148). Some authors consider that therapies such as massage, shiatsu or healing also elicit the 'relaxation response' and might thus be beneficial in similar ways.

Therapies involving touch

Many of the 'relaxing' complementary therapies involve touch. The importance of touch to physical and mental health has been demonstrated by a number of studies. Many have used an animal model and have shown that gentle caressing and stroking of young laboratory rats leads to improved weight gain, greater activity, a strengthened immune system and greater ability to withstand stress and physical damage. Studies of premature infants isolated in incubators have shown that those receiving regular physical contact in addition to regular nursery care gained weight faster, were more active, less prone to cry and had greater sensory and motor development. A trial of massage in a psychiatric setting found that a course of five daily massages reduced depression and anxiety and improved sleep.

Other therapies

A number of studies have demonstrated that the oils used by aromatherapists ('essential oils') have important medical properties. These include psychological stimulation and sedation, anti-microbial activity, effects on inflammation, pain and fever, and benefit in acne.

Spiritual healing has also been subjected to scientific scrutiny. One reviewer, Dan Benor, looked at 131 trials published in fringe journals: about 50% were positive for healing, and a number of the results were extremely dramatic indeed. However, the nature of the journals in which this research was published indicates some need for caution. There have been three well-controlled studies of healing published in peer review journals: healing was found to be significantly more effective than placebo at reducing headache pain, at calming children after stressful events and at improving general well-being in people with high blood pressure. This last study also found that people who received healing experienced greater reductions in blood pressure than

controls, though this difference was not statistically significant.

There have been no scientific trials of reflexology, shiatsu
or Feldenkrais.

In sum, though there has not been as much research on complementary healthcare as there has been on orthodox medicine,
and though we should perhaps entertain more doubt about
the claims of complementary practitioners than those of their
orthodox counterparts, there is, nonetheless, considerble
evidence to suggest that complementary therapies can provide safe and effective treatment.

2

How complementary healthcare can help people with disabilities

Complementary healthcare can help with many of the health problems of disabled people. Some of these problems, for example, sleep difficulties or recurrent infections, are also common in the non-disabled population; others, such as spasm, are more particular to disability. Listed below is a brief summary of some of the areas in which disabled people have most commonly reported benefits from complementary healthcare. Obviously, being disabled does not equate with having health problems, so you will have to decide which, if any, of these apply to you. More information on the effects of each therapy can be found in Part II.

Tension and relaxation

Many complementary therapies are particularly good at bringing about a profound sense of relaxation, something which is not only pleasant, but very health promoting (see page 155). These feelings are not restricted to the actual treatment session, they may last for several days or weeks; some people find that they are even more long-lasting: 'I'm not a tense person any more; before I was really tense'. The physical effects of relaxation can include improved sleep patterns and decreased pain and spasm.

Posture

Poor posture is very commonly improved by complementary therapies. Techniques such as Alexander training and osteopathy consciously strive to improve posture, but many people notice improved sitting, standing and walking after therapies such as massage or shiatsu. Improved posture may lead to relief from aches and pains and improved physical health.

Mobility

Mobility refers to walking, stretching, grasping and manipulating: physical disability generally involves mobility problems. Complementary therapies can sometimes improve mobility to a certain extent. Typically, people will improve on the things they are already able to do, for example, 'My walking is stronger'. It is also not uncommon for some new activities to become possible: 'I can now hold the kettle to make myself a cup of tea'.

Body perception

Many complementary therapies can help increase awareness of the body. Some people report a general feeling of being in touch with themselves; others experience more specific improvements in their perception of posture, position and movements. This can have important consequences for physical function: practitioners of complementary medicine say that using the body effectively – be it to walk, sit or hold an object – depends on our knowledge of how our body is. Body perception is sometimes called 'body image'.

Pain

There appear to be two different ways in which complementary healthcare helps with pain. Some people say that though the pain is still there, it doesn't bother them so much: the physical sensation is less unpleasant and it does not restrict their activities or enjoyment of life. Others do notice a significant decrease in the amount of pain they experience.

Recurrent infections

Complementary therapies can sometimes be effective for recurrent infections. The practitioner may try to treat such infections directly, for example, by giving a homeopathic remedy for cystitis. Alternatively, someome might notice that they had far fewer colds after a course of complementary therapy than before it, suggesting that the treatment helped strengthen their immune system.

Digestion and appetite

Many disabled people say that their appetite is better and that they enjoy food more after complementary healthcare. Many also say that their digestion is better and that eating does not cause problems such as indigestion or heartburn.

Bowels and bladder

An improvement in bowel or bladder function is one of the most commonly reported effects of complementary medicine. Problems such as diarrhoea and constipation appear particularly susceptible to complementary treatment. Many people also notice improved continence.

Spasm, Spasticity and other Involuntary Movements

Most of the complementary therapies are deeply relaxing and some people with neurological problems find that this helps to calm involuntary movements such as spasm or athetosis.

GENERAL WELL-BEING

In addition to these physical benefits, many disabled people have found that complementary healthcare has led to improved mental and emotional well-being. One of the most common phrases used is 'I feel so much better in myself'. Some people feel a sense of inner calm and peace of mind; others feel something like euphoria ('I feel bubbly'); many experience both.

Many of those who try complementary treatment also say that they feel more positive about life, that they are more confident and motivated. Common remarks are: 'I used to dwell on all the things I can't do, now I think about all the things I can' or 'I used to say "Forget it!"; now I'll give it a try.'

Some say that they have regained their sense of hope, their feeling that life is worthwhile, that there is some point to it all. Sometimes this can be quite dramatic:

> Before, everything seemed black and dismal, a bottomless pit. Now everything seems better, I find it easier to cope.

Self-image

A significant number of disabled people have problems with the image they have of their own body: they may see themselves as ugly or deformed, and, particularly where disability has been caused by accident or disease, there may be the feeling that 'My body has let me down.' There may be anger at the body, a frustration at opportunities missed because things weren't different. A counsellor for disabled people summed it up by saying: 'A large proportion of the clients I see positively hate their own body.'

There can be little doubt that many of these feelings have been engendered by a society which handicaps people whose bodies fall outside a certain norm by the emplacement of social, physical and legislative barriers and which produces a popular fiction which often associates moral weakness with physical stigma.

Improved self-image is a common consequence of complementary healthcare. One of the most commonly cited reasons for this is that many of the therapies involve touch. This touch is quite distinct from the nurse's or care worker's lifting manoeuvres, or from the physiotherapist's stretching and manipulating; it is a more gentle, human touch, one which communicates calmness and acceptance. As one massage practitioner put it:

> Sometimes I just hold the client's head or arm gently in my hands. It's a way of saying "This is how you are". You can feel when someone relaxes into it.

Another important consideration is that most complementary therapies are pleasurable and deeply relaxing. Many of the comments disabled people have made about complementary therapies make reference to how good the therapy helped them to feel:

Though I am paralysed from the waist down, Alexander lessons make me fly.

After massage I feel on top of the world.

It makes me feel wonderful.

For someone who has found their body a source of frustration, and perhaps of pain, the realization that it can also be a source of pleasure and relaxation can be profoundly important.

An associated point is that complementary healthcare can sometimes lead to an appreciation of our non-physical aspects:

Meditation put me in touch with myself. And I discovered that I was not my physical body, that I was not equal to, and bound by, this thing that other people called 'deformed'.

In addition, complementary healthcare often includes self-help. For example, in a yoga class, various postures, meditations and breathing exercises are taught for use and practice at home. Many workers have suggested that self-help improves self-image: when someone learns that they are able to help themselves, so this line of thinking goes, they feel more powerful and that they have greater worth.

Barbara Brosnan taught yoga to disabled people for many years. She says that one of the main benefits of her work was that her pupils noticed results; they could feel themselves to be changing and progressing. Moreover, no outside force could stop this process: for example, you might learn some job skill and then never get a job due to problems of access and prejudice; however, once you have learnt yoga, you can be successful by practising it at home every day.

Finally, the general approach of complementary practitioners often leads to feelings of self-worth and improved self-image. Many disabled people have incurable conditions and it is not uncommon for such individuals to be told by their doctor that because they are incurable, they are unworthy of medical attention. Many people have found the more accepting and positive attitude of complementary practitioners to have remarkable effects on their self-esteem.

COMPLEMENTARY MEDICINE AND DISABLING DISEASE

Some people become disabled as a result of diseases such as osteoarthritis, multiple sclerosis, Parkinson's disease or Friedreich's ataxia. Such individuals might benefit from complementary healthcare in some of the ways outlined above; however, there are a number of special reasons to suggest that complementary healthcare might be helpful in these conditions.

The first point is that modern medical science actually knows very little about a large number of disabling diseases. For many there is neither a cure nor treatment; what causes the diseases may be largely unknown; diagnosis is often difficult and prognoses (predictions of what will happen) are frequently impossible. It is worth remembering that whereas conventional medicine generally attempts to fight disease, complementary medicine tries to heal individuals (see page 11). If a disease is poorly understood, fighting the disease will be difficult and using a form of medicine which depends on understanding individuals rather than diseases may be more appropriate.

It is also worth pointing out that many disabling diseases exhibit a pattern of remission and relapse, which is when periods of comparatively mild symptoms alternate with periods when symptoms are more severe. This suggests that the body's susceptibility to the disease changes over time, or, to put it another way, that the body is able to resist the disease but that its ability to do so fluctuates. Practitioners of complementary medicine claim that their therapies work by stimulating the body's own self-healing and repair systems. This opens up the possibility that complementary therapies might be able to induce and maintain a remission.

Another issue worth discussing is the relationship between the mind and body in disease. Though most of the work in this area has focused on cancer, it is clearly relevant to other serious diseases. A typical study grouped women with breast cancer into four categories: 'accepters', 'deniers', 'helpless' and 'fighters'. The group with the lowest survival rates were those who passively accepted their fate; those who denied their condition did somewhat better. Those classed as 'fighters' did best of all: those women who, despite realistically accepting their diagnosis, refused to lay down and die and who continued to take an active part in their lives and treatment were those who had the longest survival times. Some authors have gone on to list what they believe to be the common characteristics of those who recover from serious disease despite great odds. Common to each of these characteristics is the willingness to change and to play an active role in healthcare.

Other workers have examined the link between stress and disease. In one experiment, laboratory rats were divided into three groups: a 'helpless' group which received electric shocks, an 'active' group which could avoid shocks by jumping over a low barrier, and a control group, which received no shocks. At the end of the experiment, the rate of cancer in the 'helpless' group was 80% higher than in the control group. This suggests that stress is linked to disease. However, the 'active' group had a rate of cancer comparable to that of the control group, and this suggests that individuals can moderate the effects of stress on their health by making an appropriate response to stressful events.

Another set of studies have linked the progress of disease to love, care and attention. One important finding is that people's immune systems are suppressed after a bereavement; immune function can also be lowered experimentally by isolating a baby monkey away from its mother. In another study, heart disease in rabbits given high doses of cholesterol was reduced by 'tender loving care', a daily session of stroking and fondling. Receiving love, care and attention makes us feel worthwhile and that life is good. This seems to help us fight serious disease.

What does all this have to do with complementary medicine? One of the problems of pointing out the link between the mind, emotions and disease is that there appears to be little you can do about it. For example, in one of their booklets, the MS Society suggests that people with multiple sclerosis should 'Think positive!' But how can you make yourself think positive? It is no more possible than forcing yourself to relax, making yourself be happy or optimistic or converting despair into a fighting spirit.

An interesting feature of complementary healthcare is that those who use it successfully often say that they now feel good about themselves, positive about life, less stressed and better able to cope. Many also say that complementary treatment has resulted in their taking a more active role in their lives and health. In other words, complementary healthcare seems to help people with serious diseases develop just those characteristics which are associated with doing well.

Different people articulate these ideas in different ways. Some like to see complementary healthcare as a 'pathway to transformation'. If you have a serious disease, that disease will become an important part of your life; you can therefore only modify your disease if you change your life. Complementary healthcare, particularly the self-help disciplines such as yoga or meditation, can help you to achieve this.

Others use the more down to earth 'wellness view of disease.' This idea is that if you cannot fight illness, your only option is to promote wellness: 'Just because the doctors can't do anything against my MS doesn't mean I can't do anything for my health.'

Another point of view is that complementary healthcare is rather like using 'spiritual jump leads'. A dispirited person – someone who feels useless, tense and defeated – is no more likely to go anywhere than a car with a flat battery and perhaps nothing is more likely to deplete the spirit than a disabling disease. Complementary healthcare can, in this view, reverse this process, helping people to feel good about themselves and about life in general.

It is clear that complementary healthcare has helped many people with disabling diseases overcome minor symptoms and improve quality of life. Whether it has affected the course of the disease can be very difficult to say; after all, who is to know what would have happened if there had been no treatment? If you have a disabling disease, you will come to your own decision as to whether complementary healthcare can help you, and if so, how and why.

You can find out more about complementary therapies and disabling disease in Part II, particularly in the sections concerning multiple sclerosis.

COMPLEMENTARY HEALTHCARE HAS OTHER ADVANTAGES

Complementary healthcare may help disabled people over-come and cope with a number of different health problems. But there is more to a treatment than its success in dealing with a specific problem. For example, someone with an arthritic condition might find that an anti-inflammatory drug and a massage might have similar short-term effects on pain. However, massage and drug therapy are essentially different forms of medicine. Drugs are generally cheap, easy to obtain and can be kept to hand; however, they can lead to unwanted side-effects and to tolerance and addiction in the long term. Massage is much safer and it is enjoyable in itself, often bringing other benefits such as improved mood and general well-being. But massage can be relatively expensive, time consuming and inconvenient. To what extent someone will use drugs or massage might depend on what importance they attach to expense and convenience compared to relaxation and freedom from side-effects.

When you think about medicine, you might want to con-sider a great deal more than the degree to which treatment might solve the particular health problems you wish to deal with. In terms of such supplementary issues, complementary healthcare might be seen to have a number of advantageous aspects.

'Positive' side-effects

Many people try complementary healthcare for some quite specific reason, for example, to improve mobility or to remedy a recurrent infection. But it is very common for such individuals to experience a number of other benefits, like feeling relaxed and more positive about life in general. The sections above on 'General well-being' and 'Self-image' discuss some of the less well defined ways in which people come to 'feel better' after complementary healthcare.

Freedom from unwanted side-effects

This well known advantage of complementary healthcare might be considered especially important for disabled people because many of their health problems are long-term and so require treatment over long periods of time. It is therefore important that any treatment has as few unwanted or harmful side-effects as possible.

Disabled people are often prescribed repeated courses of drugs to help deal with recurrent problems. Unfortunately, most drugs have side-effects and continual use can lead to problems such as tolerance, in which ever larger doses are required to achieve the same effect, and dependence, in which the body becomes so used to the drug that it cannot do without it. Sometimes, drugs can even exacerbate the problems they were meant to solve: for example, repeated doses of antibiotics can promote infection and pain killing drugs can actually add to a pain problem.

A few examples of drugs commonly prescribed to disabled people might include anti-spasmodics for someone with a spinal injury or cerebral palsy; anti-inflammatory drugs for the relief of pain from arthritis; antibiotics for recurrent urinary tract infections; anti-anxiety drugs for back pain. In each case the drugs aim to relieve troublesome symptoms. The problem is that the symptoms result from some effectively permanent condition or process, be it damage to the nervous system, damage to joints, the need for catheterization or the use of a wheelchair. So the drugs will need to be taken on an effectively permanent basis, leading to the possibility of unwanted side-effects, tolerance and dependence.

Alice, for example, has cerebral palsy and has problems with painful spasms. Her GP suggests she takes baclofen, an anti-spasmodic drug. But Alice finds that baclofen makes her woozy: 'It might dull the spasms, but it certainly dulls your mind as well'. Alice's problems with spasm will remain with her for the rest of her life, so what the doctor's advice amounts to is: 'You'll always have to dull your mind'.

What complementary healthcare might be able to offer is the control of symptoms without side-effects. Imagine that Alice learns a relaxation technique which helps to control her symptoms. It is clear that using relaxation rather than baclofen means that she can fight her pain problem without having to be, as she puts it, 'drugged senseless'.

As another example, take Giles, who has MS. He frequently experiences pain in his arms, legs and feet, but he finds that he can control these symptoms with homoeopathy. Because Giles' symptoms recur, he often has to resort to some form of medication and it is clear that it would be better for him to use homoeopathic remedies, which are generally free from unwanted side-effects, than pain-killing drugs, which make him feel drowsy and which can cause harm in the long run.

Participation, respect and individuality

Disabled people are starting to demand participation in decision making processes which affect their welfare. In addition, there have been a number of moves to encourage respect for disabled people as individuals. There are reasons to suppose that complementary healthcare is better suited to incorporate such demands than conventional medicine.

In orthodox medicine, the patient (a term which immediately suggests passivity and deference to authority) describes symptoms to a doctor. The doctor gives the patient an examination, and perhaps perform some tests. The aim is to make a diagnosis, to place the patient in a disease category. Generally speaking, all patients in the same disease category will get similar treatment. Most medical treatments, for example drugs and surgery, do not require much active participation on behalf of the patient who is merely a recipient of therapy. Moreover, patients rarely take part in the decision making process regarding which treatment should be used.

This model of treatment is often highly appropriate and its disadvantages are irrelevant in many cases. For example, if someone was knocked down by a truck and needed life-saving surgery, active participation and decision making can hardly be seen as priorities. However, for a disabled person who uses healthcare on a regular basis, such priorities may change.

One of the first things that many people notice about complementary healthcare is that they have a much more equal relationship with practitioners than in conventional medicine (see also page 232). Typical comments include: 'It was the first time I was treated as a human being rather than as an object'; 'She didn't hold power over you like a doctor would' and 'I never felt that my feelings were being respected before'. Complementary practitioners diagnose and treat individuals, rather than diseases, and many have found this to be a liberating experience:

> With the doctor, you always sense he is thinking "Here's another case of multiple sclerosis." I didn't even have to tell my acupuncturist that I had MS, I was just another person.

One of the more recent ideas in medicine is that users of health services should be given as much information as possible about their condition and their treatment. It can be disconcerting to be worked on by an 'expert' who refers to you by a term you don't understand and who uses mysterious methods you know nothing about, and for someone with a long-term health problem, this can be particularly distressing. Though there have been some remarkable improvements in communication and information provision in orthodox health services, many people have found that complementary practitioners spend more time in helping them understand treatment than their conventional counterparts.

> Instead of banging on about "clinical this" and "clinical that" and using 48 syllable words, she carefully explained to me what she was doing and why.

Terms such as 'participation' and 'empowerment' are perhaps overused and under thought about. Nevertheless, there are interesting similarities between their use amongst disabled people and their use amongst complementary practitioners. Clients of complementary healthcare are generally encouraged to participate in decision making and to take actions which promote their personal well-being.

Clients may participate in decisions concerning:

- The aim or end goal of treatent.
- Which problems require particular attention.
- The order in which treatment takes place.
- Dietary change.
- Exercises.

Actions which clients of complementary health care might take include:

- Movement and stretching exercises.
- Self-help techniques such as self-massage.

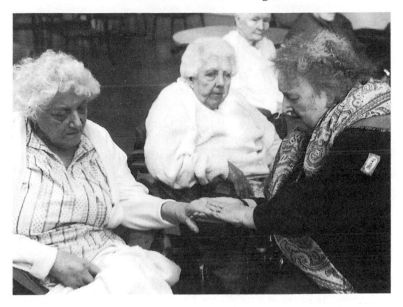

Figure 2.1 At this massage group, members are taught techniques to practise on themselves and each other.

- Relaxation, meditation and yoga.
- Dietary change.

The decision to try complementary medicine, choosing the therapy, the number of sessions wanted and how often they will be, are also active and participatory processes. Chapter 14 has further discussions of client input in complementary healthcare.

WHAT ARE THE DISADVANTAGES OF COMPLEMENTARY HEALTHCARE?

If complementary healthcare has so many advantages, why should anyone even bother seeing an orthodox doctor? It is true that many of the current problems in complementary healthcare are merely organizational; for example, a proper system of registration has not been developed for all practitioners. However, there are other disadvantages of complementary healthcare, especially when compared to conventional medicine.

Firstly, complementary healthcare often works relatively slowly and can be difficult to organize. Take the example of treatment for headache. Conventional drugs are usually effective at relieving pain and they can do so rapidly. Furthermore, they can be kept in a bottle for immediate use whenever needed. A shiatsu session might well have the same effect, but it takes longer, is much more expensive and cannot be kept to hand.

Another advantage of conventional medicine is that you can be fairly sure that treatment will work, in the short-term at least. To use the example of Alice given above, baclofen, for all its unpleasant side-effects, does usually work against spasm; meditation may or it may not.

There is good evidence to suggest that complementary therapies can have positive effects on health (see page 13). However, this does not mean that any particular treatment you receive will be of proven effectiveness. For example, there have been studies which show that herbs can remedy disease. Yet if you go to a herbalist, it is unlikely that there will have been any studies to show that the specific herbal remedy you receive is beneficial for your particular complaint.

There are also many things which complementary therapies are simply not able to do. Osteopathic treatment will not replenish blood lost from a wound; a blood transfusion is called for. Homoeopathy will not cure a joint which has been badly damaged by arthritis; a replacement joint is needed. Reflexology cannot provide a diabetic with insulin; this must be manufactured and injected.

Both complementary and conventional medicine have their advantages and disadvantages; neither can solve all health problems, each will be more appropriate in certain circumstances. It is up to every user of health services to decide which.

Summary

Complementary healthcare may be able to overcome some of the common health problems of disabled people. In addition, there are reasons to suggest that disabling diseases might be amenable to complementary treatment. But there are a number of other advantages to complementary healthcare, some of which are particularly relevant to the needs of those with disabilities: it is generally free from unwanted side-effects and the manner of treatment is one which encourages participation and emphasizes respect for individuals. However, complementary healthcare also has some disadvantages and this is why it should be seen as just one of a number of healthcare options, as complementary rather than as alternative to orthodox medicine.

3

What to expect from complementary healthcare

I have multiple sclerosis. I went to see a massage practitioner but it didn't work.

People who are considering complementary healthcare often ask: 'Does it work?' On the other hand, those who have already tried a complementary therapy are often keen to tell you whether or not it 'worked' for them. What is obvious, but apparently tends to be overlooked, is that you can only say whether something works if you have a clear idea of what happens when it does so. Does the TV work? Yes, it gives a clear picture. Does the car work? No, the engine isn't turning over. Does the sphygmomanometer work? It is clear you have to know what a sphygmomanometer does before you could answer that question.

This chapter investigates what complementary healthcare aims to do. This will not only allow you to make an informed decison on whether complementary healthcare is something you would like to try, but it will also help you assess your progress once you start. However, the best way of knowing what to expect from complementary healthcare is to read some of the examples given in Part II.

The results of complementary healthcare depend on the therapy concerned

Different therapies may aim to do very different things. Therefore what you should expect from complementary healthcare depends very much on which therapy you are trying.

Our understanding of the role and aim of a therapy is generally informed by conventional medicine. This is based upon a curative model: a person with a health problem is given a specific diagnosis describing what is wrong; the doctor aims to treat the person so that such a diagnosis can no longer be made. 'Curing', the aim of much conventional medicine, might be described as the removal of the physical manifestations of disease.

Most complementary therapies do not aim to cure; in fact, in some disciplines, practitioners can join the professional register only if they promise never to offer cures. Take the Alexander technique for example. An Alexander teacher can help you learn how to work, move and rest in an efficient way. If you have a condition such as osteoarthritis, it is clear that the Alexander technique will not cure you, yet many people with arthritis who have used the Alexander technique say that it has helped them move with less stress, tension and pain.

There are a very large number of different ways in which you can benefit from medicine. These range from 'I feel calmer', through 'My mobility is so much better' and on to 'The patient's rheumatoid factor fell by 56%'. Which particular benefit you might expect to receive depends largely on the therapy you try. Each therapy normally states its aims in its own specialized language. For example, 'Ensure a harmonious flowing of chi through the meridians' (acupuncture); 'Good use of the body' (Alexander technique) or 'The removal of the tumour without sequelae' (conventional medicine). These aims have been restated in more day-to-day language in Chapters 5–12 and you should look there for specific details.

Complementary healthcare takes time

Most practitioners of complementary healthcare believe that their techniques work by stimulating the body's own natural self-repair systems and this process, of course, takes time. Imagine an arrowhead in a wound: it is clear that removing the arrowhead will allow the wound to heal, but this still might take a number of months to happen.

One herbalist was treating a 50 year old woman who had had sleeping difficulties since she was a teenager. Two days after the first appointment, she called to complain that the herbs had not worked. The practitioner explained that you do not solve a 30 year old problem overnight and that herbs take time to act. Luckily, the client took this advice: treatment was continued and was eventually successful.

The practitioner involved says that such a reaction is very common and is a result of the widespread use of drugs. These tend to have a very rapid effect: for example, a sleeping pill will send you to sleep in about 15 minutes, a headache tablet should not take much longer than that and a steroid cream might clear up a persistent skin condition within a few days. The time needed for complementary healthcare, however, tends to be measured in weeks and months, rather than hours and days. Complementary practitioners say that this is because they treat causes rather than symptoms. In the case of a sleep difficulty, taking a sleeping pill or tranquillizer will cure one symptom: not being able to get to sleep on one particular night. Tackling the underlying problem, be it anxiety, pain or whatever, is a much greater task and will take much longer.

How long it will take for you to resolve a particular health problem, and how many sessions with a practitioner you will need, depends very much on what problems you have and how long you have had them. As a general guideline, most people start to see some effect before the sixth session. Many therapies come to some kind of completion after 12 to 15 sessions, but this figure might be two or three times that for serious or long-term problems. Often, a period of quite intense treatment, say once or twice a week for a couple of months, will be followed by quarterly or twice-yearly 'top-up' visits.

These general rules are often broken when disability is involved. One of the common words used to describe the role of complementary therapies in the healthcare of disabled people is 'management'. This reflects the view that problems recur if not regularly addressed. For example, one woman with MS found that reflexology helped her bladder problems enormously, but she also noticed that if she missed a few treatments, she started having trouble once more.

Perhaps the reason for this is that in disability, the 'underlying problem' may not, in fact, be treatable. For example,

James, who has cerebral palsy, has regular shiatsu treatments and this helps him with a number of problems such as pain and poor sleep. However, a significant element in these problems appears to be his use of a wheelchair and his athetosis (involuntary writing motions), neither of which can be changed by shiatsu treatment.

In summary, it takes time for changes to take place in complementary healthcare, particularly if problems are long-standing. For some disabled people, regular treatment may be necessary to ensure that improvements are maintained.

'Miracle cures'

Media coverage of complementary medicine seems almost exclusively concerned with miracles and miracle cures. In the case of spiritual healing, this perception is so ingrained that most people believe it to be all-or-nothing: the healer lays on hands and either the client immediately leaps out of the wheelchair or nothing happens at all.

Dr Peter May, a member of the General Synod of the Church of England and a Southampton GP, has studied claims of miraculous healing for 20 years. By careful study of the medical records, he has exposed a number of the most celebrated cases as somewhat less than miracles. He says this of his work:

> As a Christian, I do not doubt God's healing power. But my experience teaches me that when He answers prayers, He normally respects the integrity of the created order . . . He does not change dogs into cats.

A non-religious way of putting this might be that, though the healing powers of the mind and body are remarkable, they are not unlimited. In certain cases, people may make improvements which are unlikely from an orthodox point of view, for example, a person with cancer being alive and well many years after a prediction that they would be dead within months. But no-one will make an improvement which breaks the laws of nature.

The effects of complementary healthcare can sometimes be very dramatic. In the odd rare case, a practitioner can indeed provide rapid and dramatic relief, and, given the fact that many thousands of practitioners give many millions of consultations every year, this is perhaps not unexpected. But this is not the common experience of people who try complementary therapies.

Perhaps, most important of all, many practitioners believe that the people who look for miracles tend to be those who benefit least from complementary healthcare. The reason for this is simple: playing an active role and taking on responsibility is an important part of complementary healthcare; looking for miracles means lying back and letting some outside agent do the work.

SPECIFIC AND NON-SPECIFIC EFFECTS OF
COMPLEMENTARY HEALTHCARE

John went to see an osteopath because he had a painful back. After a few sessions, his back was free of pain and felt much more flexible. Ruth decided to treat herself to a course of massage treatments. The massage left her feeling calm and relaxed and she found it much easier to cope with hassles at the office.

John experienced what is known as a specific effect of therapy, when a particular symptom or health problem improves. Ruth, on the other hand, experienced non-specific or generalized effects: though she 'feels better' in herself, she finds it difficult to point to individual symptoms which no longer worry her.

Conventional medicine tends to concentrate on specific effects. For example, a doctor might treat athlete's foot with an anti-fungal skin cream. The aim in this case is very specific: to eradicate the fungus and thereby relieve the symptoms of pain and itching.

Complementary therapies are found at the opposite end of the spectrum. Almost everyone who tries a therapy says that they feel 'better in themselves' or that they have a 'general sense of well-being'. Often, however, they may find it difficult to identify the exact way in which they feel better and specific health problems may be left unchanged.

Within complementary healthcare, different therapies vary as to the degree to which their effects are specific or generalized. Massage, healing, meditation and tai chi are good examples of techniques where the outcome of treatment is generalized; acupuncture, osteopathy and homoeopathy are examples of therapies which have more specific effects. There is much crossover however. People who have successful osteopathic treatment often experience an improved sense of well-being; conversely massage, and even yoga and meditation, can be used for specific symptoms.

It is important to discuss the difference between specific and non-specific effects of treatment. When many people ask the question: 'What will complementary healthcare do for me?' they often expect the answer to be in terms of improved physical function, recovery from illness or the reversal of a degenerative disease (i.e. specific effects of treatment). It is often seen as somehow weak and irrelevant if an answer is given in terms of more generalized effects, for example, feelings of well-being and self-esteem or better coping with pain. Perhaps the reason for this is that we are brought up with conventional medicine, and conventional medicine often places greater emphasis on

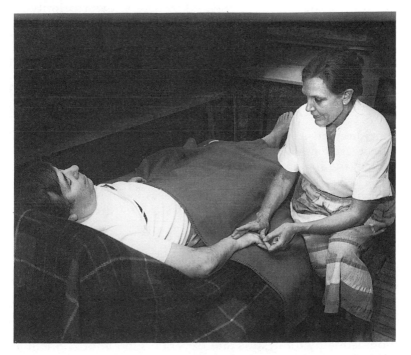

Figure 3.1 Complementary healthcare often leads to feelings of relaxation and calmness.

physical changes than on how people feel. However, there is no reaosn why this should be so. First of all, what we live with on a day-to-day basis is just as much our feelings about ourselves and our lives as our physical state. Secondly, the effects a certain physical condition will have on our lives often depends on our mental and emotional adjustment to that condition. Perhaps the best example of this is chronic pain: some people who have long-term pain cope with their condition by using a variety of physical and mental exercises. Though the actual degree of pain they experience may be little changed, the effects it has on their lives, such as preventing employment or interfering with social activities, will be greatly reduced.

Interestingly, what many disabled people have pointed out first about their experiences of complementary healthcare were the general effects of treatment, their feeling of well-being, relaxation and motivation. Specific improvements in mobility or function have often appeared to take a lower priority.

Examples of the effects of complementary healthcare

Specific effects	Non-specific effects
Stronger walking	General feelings of well-being
Increased joint mobility	'The pain is still there, but it doesn't bother me so much'
Improved speech	Relaxation, calmness and
Decreased swelling	improved sleep
Recovery from infection	Increased motivation; feeling positive about life
Improved bowel and bladder function	'I feel in touch with myself'

COMPLEMENTARY HEALTHCARE IS NOT ALWAYS SUCCESSFUL

Sometimes, a course of complementary treatment does not result in any significant benefit. Though complementary therapy may fail altogether (for example, a person might try homoeopathy for cystitis and experience no improvement at all) it is perhaps more common for an individual to gain some sort of benefit, though not enough to make the time and expense of healthcare worthwhile. For example, someone might find that reflexology makes him feel very relaxed and well in himself for a few hours after each session, but after a number of treatments he may realize that he has experienced only marginal relief from some of his most troublesome symptoms.

It is not unusual for a person to try a number of different practitioners and therapies before finding a combination which works for them (see also page 57). You should not expect complementary healthcare always to be successful. Your own experiences may well be mixed, with perhaps some of the things you try not being fully worth the time, money and effort you may have invested in them.

THE EFFECTS OF MEDICAL CHARACTERISTICS

A number of different factors affect the success of complementary treatment. This section looks at the effects of what might be termed the medical characteristics of a client on the outcome of treatment. These are age, disease duration (how long someone has had a particular health problem before coming to the practitioner), the severity of the symptoms and the existence of structural damage or deformity (for example, large-scale joint erosion in arthritis).

Complementary practitioners say that these factors do affect what happens in treatment, but they do so in a special way. Specific effects of treatment, such as improved mobility, do depend largely on the medical characteristics; non-specific effects, such as relaxation, are entirely independent of such factors.

Complementary healthcare can improve a person's general sense of well-being regardless of their medical condition. Perhaps the ultimate example of this is the use of complementary therapies with people who are dying. Massage practitioners and healers commonly visit hospices and it is said that their work helps improve the quality of life of those who are facing death.

Many disabled people have a condition which will not be improved by any form of medical intervention. Yet many of these have gained great benefit from complementary healthcare. There are numerous examples throughout this book where individuals have experienced an increased feeling of general well-being without any specific 'medical' change taking place. Joe, for example, had a stroke. He says that acupuncture left him feeling much better in himself, though it did not affect his mobility in any way or clear up any other particular major problems. In fact, if a doctor had examined Joe before and after the acupuncture treatment, she might well have reported that no changes had taken place.

Specific effects of complementary therapies for disabled people might include: increased mobility; changes in the rate of disease progression; decreased pain and control of recurrent infections. Complementary practitioners say that their ability to facilitate such changes does depend, in part, on the client's age, the duration of the disease, the severity of the symptoms and the existence or structural damage. Though there are no hard and fast rules – most practitioners have cases where an elderly person made a dramatic improvement or where an individual recovered from a disabling disease of many years' duration – it is possible to discern the following trends.

Age

Practitioners of complementary healthcare believe that healing takes place by stimulating the body's own regenerative mechanisms. This self-healing ability is reduced as a person gets older: great functional improvements are much less common among older people than amongst the younger or middle aged.

Disease duration

For almost all forms of medicine, the adage, 'The sooner treatment starts, the better' is appropriate. Generally speaking, the longer an individual has had a disease, the more difficult it will be for a practitioner to reverse the progress of that disease. Practitioners who have treated conditions such as MS or rheumatoid arthritis say that if they work with someone within the first seven or eight years of their diagnosis, improvements are often marked. After that period of time, it can be much more difficult to affect the course of the disease.

Similarly, people who have had a stroke appear to receive the most benefit if treatment starts within six months.

Symptom severity

In general, the milder the symptoms, the easier they are to control.

Structural damage

There are some structural changes that no practitioner will be able to remedy. For example, complementary medicine will obviously not make an amputated limb regrow. In rheumatic and arthritic conditions, joints may become damaged as the disease progresses. Most complementary practitioners say that they will not be able to reverse this damage, though some say that if the body stays healthy enough, long enough, repair of bony structures may be possible. In neurological conditions such as MS or stroke, complementary healthcare will not heal dead or scarred nerve tissue. However, because there is no exact correlation between the degree of damage to the nervous system and the degree of disability, it is difficult to assess what level of functioning it might be possible for any particular individual to recover.

In general, it is very difficult to know what any individual's potential might be. Doctors have frequently been criticized for setting out what degree of progress is statistically most likely and pouring cold water on their patients' expectations if they exceed their own. Complementary healthcare is about maximizing individual well-being and potential: it is not about predicting what that might be. Once it is understood that instant miracle cures are not on offer, and that certain factors can make progress more difficult, it is up to the individual to decide what he or she wants and expects from healthcare.

Summary

What you should expect from complementary therapy depends, at least partly, on the therapy you are trying. This is because different therapies may have very different aims. One thing you should expect is for complementary healthcare to take time: effects are generally noticed in weeks and months, rather than hours and days.

The benefits of complementary healthcare can be either non-specific (for example, a general feeling of well-being), or specific (for example, reduced frequency of infections or stronger walking). Though complementary healthcare almost always results in some form of non-specific benefit, the ability of a therapy to bring about a specific effect is affected by the medical characteristics of the client, for example, their age and the severity of the symptoms. Finally, complementary therapy is not always successful. Some people have to try a variety of therapies and practitioners before finding a combination which suits them; others do not experience significant benefit.

4

How to decide on complementary healthcare

People who are considering complementary healthcare often worry about quackery: they wonder how they can be sure that a practitioner is competent or that a therapy is safe and effective. But deciding on complementary healthcare is actually a two-stage process. Firstly, you do have to ask: 'Are the therapy and practitioner safe and reputable and do I have a reasonable chance of success?' But you also have to decide: 'Are the therapy and practitioner right for me?' Making decisions about complementary healthcare is not merely a case of avoiding quacks; it is also about positive choices of what you really want from healthcare and a means by which you can maximize your chance of success.

In this respect, complementary healthcare is little different from other decisions you have to make. Take, for example, going on a holiday. Firstly, you have to make sure that your tour operator is reputable and that they won't take your money and send you to a half-built hotel, or one without wheelchair access if that is what you paid for. You also have to make sure that your destination isn't being ravaged by disease or civil war. But once you are sure that your holiday is basically safe and sound, you will still want to consider where it is you want to go and what it is you really want to do.

The basic question of how to make sure that a practitioner and therapy are safe and reputable will be considered first. The discussion will then focus on the importance of personal preference in making decisions about complementary healthcare.

WHICH THERAPIES ARE SAFE AND EFFECTIVE?

This question is answered by the contents of Part II. Though decisions about the value of a therapy will always be somewhat subjective, the criteria used for the purposes of this book are listed below. Though not every therapy listed in Part II fulfils every criterion, each fulfils at least a significant number.

Tradition and progress

Most of the therapies have traditions spanning at least a hundred years. What is perhaps more important is that during this time the therapy has progressed. Increasing numbers of people are practising the therapy or expressing an interest in it; practitioners are opening new areas of work; scientific understanding and validation is increasing; acceptance is increasing.

Safety

All the therapies included can be considered to be relatively safe forms of healthcare, where practised by competent professionals.

Interest from the medical profession

Though many members of the medical profession are suspicious of complementary healthcare, a large number of doctors, nurses, physiotherapists etc. are developing an interest in, and even practising, complementary therapies. Few are using therapies other than those mentioned in the main text of this book.

Scientific validation

Many complementary therapies have been subject to scientific evaluation (see page 13). Of those included in the book, all but a few have some form of scientific validation. Some of those which are not mentioned in the main text have failed under scientific scrutiny.

Homoeopathy and crystal healing:
an example comparison

In a tradition spanning more than 150 years, many thousands of homoeopaths have had successful practices in many different countries worldwide. Large numbers of conventionally qualified doctors practise homoeopathy and its use is being increasingly accepted within the medical community. Moreover, a number of scientific studies have shown homoeopathy to be safe and effective.

The only criterion which crystal healing fulfils is that of safety: of course, crystal healers will say that their therapy is good for you and they can probably also tell you a few successful case histories, but then so would any practitioner.

The therapies covered in the main text of this book are what might be described as the mainstream of complementary healthcare. Each is safe and gives you a reasonable chance of success and it is suggested that if you want to try a complementary therapy, you would be best off trying one of the ones listed in Part II.

HOW DO I FIND A REPUTABLE PRACTITIONER?

Avoiding quacks is probably one of the major concerns of anyone considering complementary healthcare. One of the problems is that absolutely anyone can call themselves a complementary practitioner, no matter what their training, so if you look in the phone book under say, 'homoeopathy', you have no way of telling whether the individuals listed are competent and qualified to practise.

What can make matters worse is that practitioners sometimes give themselves titles such as 'Member of the Licentiate of Homoeopathy', 'Doctor of Alternative Medicine', 'Diploma in Reflexology' or 'MFHom'. Some of these titles are meaningless and they can mislead people into believing that a practitioner has a worthy qualification when this may not in fact be so.

Luckily, finding a reputable practitioner is a task made considerably easier by the existence of professional registers. In some therapies, a governing body has managed to establish broad agreement on what skills and knowledge are needed to

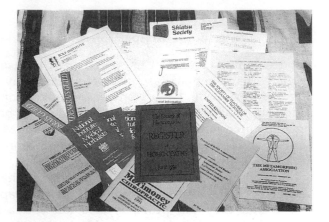

Figure 4.1 Professional registers can be a useful resource for anyone trying to locate a competent practitioner of complementary healthcare.

practise the therapy competently. Individuals meeting standards set out by the governing body are placed on a register and members of the public can then use this register to find capable practitioners. Some organizations have computerized registers and can give you names and addresses over the phone; others can send you a printed copy of their register by post.

One organization which holds a register for a number of different therapies is the Institute for Complementary Medicine (see also page 276). The British Register of Complementary Practitioners, as it is known, has been well thought out. However, at the time of writing, the number of practitioners on the register is relatively small, so though this is a useful resource, it is certainly not a cure all.

Unfortunately, some therapies do not have a single governing body and so either there is no register at all, or there are many, each with different requirements. Where there is no broad agreement on standards, there is no easy way to tell who is a competent practitioner and who is not. There are some qualifications which are worth watching for, many of which are barely worth the paper they are written on and, regardless, many excellent practitioners advertise no qualifications at all.

The therapies for which finding a practitioner may not be a simple case of checking a register are as follows: massage, aromatherapy, reflexology, hypnotherapy, nutrition and disciplines such as meditation, yoga and tai chi. Registers do exist for each of these (see the relevant chapters in Part II) but these registers either fail to include some competent practitioners or fail to set high enough standards. These registers might be seen as a useful source of appropriate contacts rather than as means of guaranteeing therapeutic competence. The advice given below on where to look for a practitioner and how to check whether a practitioner is reputable refers primarily to these therapies.

If you are not using a register, good ways to find a practitioner include recommendations from friends and colleagues, asking your GP, contacting natural health centres, asking for information at a local health store and contacting a registered practitioner of a different therapy. So, for example, you could find the name of your local osteopath from the register of osteopaths and ask if they know of a good local massage practitioner. Bad places to look for practitioners include natural healing fairs and festivals, magazines and newspapers and anything that resembles 'hawking', such as leaflets under the door, mail shots or direct approaches in person or by phone. Yellow Pages can sometimes be a help, but, of course, anyone can get themselves listed. Massage, for example, is found on the same page as 'Meat Markets', something which is perhaps appropriate given that a majority of the listings include pictures of big breasted girls claiming to offer 'exclusive services'.

How to check unregistered practitioners

If you are interested in trying a therapy which does not have a widely recognized register, you cannot be sure that any practitioner you contact will be competent and you will have to make sure of this yourself. This is not as scary or difficult as it sounds: you merely have to ask a few questions and watch out for a few danger signs.

It can be a good idea to arrange to meet practitioners for an interview or just have a chat to them on the phone. They might also send or give you some literature. Things to be on the alert for are as follows.

Guarantees of successful results Every responsible practitioner knows that the healing cannot be guaranteed, simply because people are not predictable and no medicine is 100% effective. In general, the more a practitioner promises, the less he or she will be able to provide.

Promises of specific cures for specific conditions 'One 15 minute session of magnet therapy will help cure your arthritis' is a good example of a quack claim. Compare it to something which would be perfectly acceptable, say an osteopath telling you: 'I have been quite successful at treating low back pain in the past and I think osteopathy might actually be quite good for your problem'.

Promises that your entire life will be made right A classic trick of quacks and cults is to delude that they have the answer to all your problems: 'Madame Lako can help you overcome all life's difficulties and sorrows'.

Advertising It is one thing for practitioners to put their card up in the village newsagent or in the health store. It is something else to put an advert in a magazine or newspaper, or to put a card through the door. Hawking for business is definitely something you find more amongst quacks than amongst reputable practitioners.

Propaganda 'I can cure the world and everyone should try my therapy and no-one else, especially not doctors, knows what they are talking about'.

Prying or bullying attitude It is a bad sign if a practitioner asks for irrelevant details or seems to take a vicarious delight in finding out about your life. If this happens, ask the practitioner why he or she needs to know a particular fact (after all, you can't be sure it is irrelevant). Bullying is out: 'You really ought to do what I say, Mrs Jones, what on earth is the matter with you?'

Unsolicited offers of therapy If someone you don't know approaches you and offers any kind of healing service, refuse: 'When my brother was dying of cancer, he was approached by all sorts of healers, quacks and weirdos. They took his money, raised false hopes and robbed him of the chance to come to terms with his death. It was like vultures hovering over a corpse'.

Mystical language People who use unusual and irregular language generally have something to hide or, at the very least, they want to confuse you out of making an informed judgement. Take: 'A healing experience with starlight elixirs. Using celestial energy and love channels . . . ' and compare this to 'The Alexander technique teaches us to use ourselves more effectively in daily life'. Some good practitioners and therapies do use rather unusual language though, so don't rule anyone out on this criterion alone.

Asking questions

If there are no immediate danger signals, it can be a good idea to go on and ask your practitioner a few basic questions. If you are embarrassed about this, tell your practitioner that you just want to make sure: a good practitioner will understand. The questions you might consider asking are:

- What methods of treatment do you use and what do they involve?
- When, where and for how long were you trained?
- How long have you been practising?
- Can you suggest any other therapies, including conventional ones?
- Would you be prepared to refer me elsewhere?
- Do you have professional indemnity insurance?

If access is a problem for you ask:

- Is your practice accessible? Can you do outcalls?

There are no set 'correct' answers, though a practitioner should have indemnity insurance and should not have been trained exclusively through a correspondence course. What you should look out for is the way in which the questions are answered. It is a good sign if the practitioner answers your questions calmly and openly; bluster, confusing answers and 'propaganda' (see above) are bad signs. The good rule of thumb is: 'the more a practitioner promises, the less they will be able to provide', so avoid any practitioners who spout on about how completely brilliant they are, what good training they had and how there is going to be absolutely no need to refer you elsewhere.

Despite all that has been said, there is no need to be suspicious of everyone. Bear in mind that making a wrong decision is unlikely to lead to disaster, especially if you follow the advice in Chapter 14 about what should not happen during treatment.

PERSONAL PREFERENCE IN DECISIONS ABOUT COMPLEMENTARY HEALTHCARE

In conventional medicine, decisions about treatment are normally left up to the doctor. There is a good reason for this: only someone with medical training can be expected to understand which orthodox therapy is most appropriate for a particular diagnosis.

When some people try complementary healthcare, they expect decisions about treatment to be taken off their hands in a similar way. They commonly ask: 'I have condition X, which complementary therapy is the best for me?' or even: 'I have condition X and someone suggested yoga. Which type of yoga should someone with condition X try?'

Complementary healthcare is all about treating people, not diseases. Decisions about treatment should therefore be about people, not diseases. In other words, what complementary therapies someone should try, and which practitioner they should visit, is a matter of that person's individual preference. It is not something that can be dictated or prescribed depending on a medical diagnosis.

There are, of course, some guidelines. Certain groups of therapies do seem more appropriate to certain types of problems than others (see Chapter 5). But it is worth remembering that different types of complementary healthcare offer very different things. If you ask someone whether you should have a snack, a cup of tea or a lie down, they would probably ask you whether you were hungry, thirsty or sleepy. In a similar way if you asked someone to tell you whether you should go for masssage, take up yoga or try acupuncture, the best response would not be for them to choose a therapy for you, but to ask what you really wanted from complementary healthcare and to explain what each therapy offered.

The second reason why personal preference is so important in deciding about complementary healthcare, is that whether a treatment is successful or not often depends on whether the person receiving that treatment believes that it can work. The best example of this is what doctors call the 'placebo effect', which is when patients improve after receiving a pill containing no active medicine (a placebo). The placebo effect suggests that a person's faith in a treatment can have therapeutic benefits, and studies of the placebo effect have shown that placebo pills have about a 30% success rate in treating pain. Other studies have demonstrated that very large and very small pills work better than those of medium size; that two pills work better than one; that red pills are more effective than those of other colours and that injections work best of all, especially if they sting. The fact that individuals' belief in their treatment influences whether they get well is taken so seriously by the medical profession that every drug has to be tested against a placebo to prove that it works.

A cancer doctor in the USA called Bernie Segal has noticed a similar, but opposite effect. Segal asks his patients to draw pictures of themselves receiving treatment and often, where a patient's treatment is not going well, he will find that they have drawn a negative image. For example, chemotherapy is drawn as the devil with a poisonous injection, and radiotherapy might be seen as a death ray from an alien machine.

So a person's attitude towards his or her therapy can affect whether or not it is successful. This means that anyone deciding on healthcare can maximize their chance of success by ensuring that their attitude towards the therapy they choose will be better rather than worse. This doesn't mean that somehow you must force yourself to pledge blind allegiance to whatever course of treatment you choose; what it means is that you should choose a therapy that strikes a chord with you, something which you find appealing, and that you should seek out a practitioner with whom you could form a positive and therapeutic relationship. Choosing the therapy and practitioner you feel suits you is an important way of ensuring that you have the best possible chance of benefitting from complementary healthcare.

Choosing a therapy

It's no good dragging someone who is frightened of needles, kicking and screaming, to the acupuncture clinic. Firstly, they will probably not enjoy it; secondly, it probably won't do much good. On the other hand, it is simply not true that, as some conventional practitioners have claimed: 'Homoeopathy may help those who believe in it . . . healing is for those that have faith'.

Practitioners of complementary healthcare do not demand specific beliefs from their clients. They point out that animals and children can be treated with complementary therapies and say that this proves that you are not required to have faith in complementary medicine to be successfully treated. But practitioners do ask that clients have an open mind, and trying a therapy you are scared of, or one you think is quackery, is unlikely to lead to an open mind or a successful treatment.

The next step in choosing a therapy is deciding what you really want from healthcare. For example, are you looking for something relaxing and soothing? Is pain a problem? Is a recurrent urinary tract infection your most worrying symptom? Or are you seeking greater awareness of your mind and body? Determining your priorities will help you cut down the list of therapies you could try but this is not as easy as it sounds. It is not uncommon for people to 'feel like trying complementary medicine' without really knowing what they hope to achieve.

When you are thinking about what you want from healthcare, it is important to think about what you might want in general from your life, as well as thinking about specific health problems such as a painful knee or poor sleep. For example, do you want to do something in which you can go out and meet other people? Do you want something you can practice at home and incorporate into your daily life? Is one-to-one care and attention important to you? Are you interested in seeing how you could change your life to maximize your well-being? Would you like to use complementary healthcare to take you off in new directions, to learn new philosophies or achieve spiritual satisfaction? Or do you positively not want any of these things?

The third thing to consider as you read through the therapies in Part II is your basic gut feeling towards each of them. Do any therapies particularly attract you? Do you like the ideas behind one of the therapies or think you might enjoy some of the techniques involved? Choosing something that strikes a chord with you will not only mean you will enjoy treatment more, it will increase your chances of success.

For example, one inner London health clinic which provides a range of complementary healthcare has large numbers of clients from the local West Indian community. Workers at the clinic noticed that these clients tended to do better with herbal medicine than homoeopathy and when they asked why this might be the case, they were told that there was a strong tradition of herbal medicine in West Indian culture and that it was something they could understand and associate with. For another example, take the case of Phyllis and Christine on page 238; Christine, who had personally chosen Alexander technique, had a very much more successful treatment than Phyllis, who went for metamorphic technique because 'they told me to'.

The final thing to say about choosing a therapy is that it can be difficult to get it right first time.

> I had shoulder pain following an accident and I thought that acupuncture would be the best treatment. It was okay, but the effects didn't last long. After a bit, I switched to a cranial osteopath. She was great! The treatment was terrific and I am much better now.

One of the reasons for this is that there appears to be a natural variation in how individuals respond to different therapies. It just might be the case that, for reasons no-one can explain, one particular therapy might be more appropriate for you than another. Practitioners often make comments such as: 'Reflex zone therapy just happens to suit some people more than others', and such variation can sometimes actually be measured. There is a special scale which rates 'hypnotizability' and, similarly, homoeopaths engaged in scientific trials often divide their patients up into different groups depending on how well they fit the prescribing signs for their homoeopathic remedy.

Though avoiding therapies you fear or doubt, considering what it is you really want from healthcare and choosing a therapy based on your own intuitive judgement will give you the best chance of hitting on the most appropriate therapy first time, there will always be unknown factors and a process of trial and error is sometimes the only way of finding the health practice that will be most effective for you.

Choosing the right practitioner

It is essential that any practitioner you choose has the minimum basic qualifications to practice his or her therapy competently (see 'How do I find a reputable practitioner?' above). But there is more to choosing a practitioner than checking qualifications.

There is wide agreement in complementary healthcare that the relationship between client and practitioner has a greater effect on the outcome of treatment than any other single factor. This means that you will very much increase your chances of success if you make attempts to find a practitioner with whom you can form a positive and rewarding relationship. Some workers have used the phrase 'The Therapeutic Partnership' to describe such a relationship. This suggests that both practitioner and client play an equal, if distinct, role in the enterprise of helping the client achieve greater well-being and that an individual should choose a practitioner with the same care as they choose any other partner.

A number of studies on counselling and psychotherapy have supported the idea that finding the right practitioner should come before other considerations, such as which therapy you prefer. Briefly, the findings have been that the effectiveness of counselling depends not so much on the particular technique used, nor even on whether the counsellor was fully trained or not, but on whether the client finds that the practitioner possesses characteristics such as genuineness, empathy, understanding and warmth.

Finding the right practitioner, like finding a marital partner, is something that will always depend ultimately on personal choice. But there are some pointers to what you should look for. When considering any practitioner, you might ask yourself a number of questions:

- Do you trust the practitioner and have faith in his or her integrity, honesty and ability?
- Do you feel that you could confide in the practitioner?
- Do you feel that you could form an equal relationship with this practitioner or do you sense that he or she would wield power over you?
- Would the practitioner be prepared to admit 'I don't know' or acknowledge weaknessess in knowledge or skills?
- Will the practitioner suggest self-care or refer you to other practitioners if the need arose? Or do you think that the practitioner might monopolize your healthcare so as to retain power and sole credit?
- Will the practitioner help you set your own goals and agenda; or will this practitioner try to impose his or her own goals upon you?
- Do you feel the practitioner will treat you with respect and dignity?
- Does the practitioner make you feel hopeful and strengthen your expectations that you can be helped?
- Would you prefer the practitioner to be of a certain gender or age? Is the practitioner's cultural background important to you?

Of course, all that has been written is very much 'in an ideal world'. For example, your choice of practitioners might be limited by where you live, how much money you have or, if transport or access is a problem, which practitioners are prepared to do outcalls. You might also find that certain practitioners are booked up and can take on no more clients.

You might ask how it is you can come to meet a practitioner before considering a course of treatment. Some authors have suggested some kind of pre-treatment interview, in which practitioner and client can get to know each other and make a decision as to whether they should consider a course of therapy. Though such an interview is a fairly standard routine in counselling, it does not appear to be widely practical for other therapies. A brief chat on the phone is one excellent way of making an assessment of a potential practitioner: you could, for example, ask a few questions about the therapy and whether it could help for your health problem and take the opportunity to discuss fees and outcalls. Even a few minutes chat can give you a clue as to whether you could work with a practitioner. Advice from friends and collegues can also be useful.

However, you might only be able to decide how you feel about a practitioner after a few sessions. It can be annoying, embarrassing and expensive to change practitioners once a course of treatment has actually begun. But if you have a problem you really want solved, and if you see healthcare as a long-term enterprise, it may be the best option.

Finally, don't worry unduly about finding a suitable practitioner. It is also worth pointing out that your relationship with your practitioner becomes less crucial in situations when that relationship cannot be close, for example, if you only want gentle massage once in a while, or if you want to learn a discipline such as yoga.

Other considerations

Access is a vital issue for many disabled people and you will obviously have to rule out any practitioners who don't do outcalls if their place of work is inaccessible to you. If you have problems finding a practitioner purely because of access difficulties, it is worth challenging one of the inaccessible practitioners you have contacted and asking what they think their profession is about and whether they feel that disabled people should be excluded. Appealing to a practitioner's higher nature can work wonders.

A number of other issues might also influence your choice of practitioner and therapy. These include: how far you have to travel, where you have to travel to, how convenient the times are and, of course, money.

Many people think that such things should be ignored: 'It's my health isn't it. I don't care how far I have to go, what I have to do or how much I have to pay!' The problem is that such considerations can exert subtle influences on the outcome of treatment. Imagine you do something you don't want to in order to get treated; for example, you might have to travel for a long time. It is possible that because you subconsciously associate visiting the practitioner with something unpleasant (the travelling) you might sub-consciously want treatment to be unsuccessful so as to avoid it.

It might sound a little far fetched, but this is how many psychologists look at the mind. There is also some evidence that, in the case of counselling at least, people who travel more than 20 minutes to see a practitioner tend to have less success.

So though each of the people below might appear to be making important decisions on trivial grounds, there is definitely some sense in the choices they make.

> I had a choice between two osteopaths, one of whom worked at the Sports Centre. I find it such a depressing place I chose the other one.

> I decided on a practitioner who lived near the heath so I could go for a walk afterwards.

> It was a case of choosing the practitioner who was free in the times that most suited me.

'There's nothing wrong with not "doing" complementary medicine'

Some people feel pressured to try complementary healthcare. It is not uncommon for friends to repeatedly mention therapies they've heard about ('A colleague of Mrs D has taken her daughter and its had the most amazing effects') and the implicit and often unwanted suggestion is that 'you too should try it'. Simply reading about complementary health care – this book, for example – can often have a similar effect.

Another prevalent assumption is that it is incumbent upon a person with a health problem to explore every avenue and leave no stone unturned etc. etc. in the quest for health. Also, in some social groups, there can be a strange form of inverted snobbery about healthcare: people who try alternative medicine are seen as adventurous and empowered, whereas those who stick to staid and boring conventional medicine are, well, staid and boring and conventional.

The comment which forms the title of this section was made by the mother of a disabled child. She said that she has met many parents who spend years taking their child off to dozens of different therapists. She says that these parents often forget, understandably, that there is more to life than therapy, and that time and effort can also be spent profitably on just playing with and getting to know a child. Moreover, spending a high proportion of time in medical contexts can reinforce individuals' perception of themselves as different, as sick and disabled.

In short, there shouldn't be any 'shoulds' about complementary healthcare. You might well read this book and feel that complementary healthcare was not something you would be interested in pursuing. If you feel your time would be better spent sitting in the sun than lying on a treatment couch, then all well and good; nevertheless, be aware that you may sometimes feel under pressure to change your mind.

GROUP SITUATIONS

The most common healthcare groups are self-help groups, run by and for people with similar health problems. Sometimes, self-help groups are for people who care for those with a certain health problem, for example, parents with disabled children. Such self-help groups are widely recognized to be valuable and helpful. For information on how to find an appropriate health group, see the resources listing on page 276.

The concern here, however, is when complementary healthcare takes place in groups. The majority of examples of complementary healthcare used throughout this book involve a client and practitioner in a one-to-one situation. But this need not always be the case: yoga, tai chi and meditation are usually taught to groups; other therapies which can sometimes take place with more than one client include massage, healing, counselling and the Alexander technique.

Group healthcare can take a number of different forms. The massage classes taught at some day centres usually consist of about 10 to 15 clients and one or two practitioners. Such classes typically involve three stages: initial warm-up stretches, massage and a period of relaxation. A prominent aspect of these classes is self-help. The clients are often taught simple techniques of self-massage along with stretches and relaxation, techniques intended for use outside the class as well as during it. Other possibilities for the massage period include each client getting a short (10–15 minute) massage from a practitioner and clients working in pairs, with the practitioner demonstrating a technique and the client practising it on a partner. Similar classes are run by Adult Education Institutes in many areas and may include reflexology and shiatsu, as well as massage.

At healing centres, a number of healers will work together in one room with clients waiting together, and relaxing afterwards, as a group. The actual practice of the healing remains one-on-one, but the group context, and the fact that you do not have your own practitioner, makes the experience very different from private contact with an individual healer. Healing is also sometimes taught through adult education.

Another alternative is for everyone in the group to experience therapy at the same time. In groups for counselling or art therapy, everyone participates and is involved, to a greater or lesser degree, throughout the session. In some healing groups, everyone gives and receives healing and there may be some group healing exercises.

What are the advantages and disadvantages of group situations? Some people prefer groups purely for the social element and see getting out of the house and meeting people to be an end in itself. Group work is also much cheaper than individual sessions. But there are also some more subtle benefits of working in groups. Some people find the sense of mutual support and shared problems to be very rewarding. Groups can help break the 'I am the only sick and lonely person in the world' syndrome and some disabled people have found working in groups with the able-bodied to be a liberating experience. Such situations can usefully break the old stereotype of disabled people as sick and crippled and in need of help and the able-bodied as super-fit providers of care.

An associated point is that, in supportive group environment, people can try out new roles. For example, an individual at a massage class could try out being the giver of care and comfort, perhaps reversing a normal role of being its recipient. And because groups are social situations, people can try out social roles too, for example, initiating activity, being assertive or on the other hand, letting others take the lead.

Some people prefer group situations because they are less intense than one-on-one contact with a practitioner. A slight variation is that visiting a practitioner can be seen as decreasing self-reliance. One client has said that she wanted to avoid solo visits to a practitioner because, now that she had MS, she didn't want to depend on anyone but herself.

Disadvantages to working in groups include less individual attention, less chance of building up a relationship with a practitioner and, possibly, problems connected with confidentiality: it can be more difficult to talk about personal problems to a group than an individual practitioner. Another point is that groups practising complementary healthcare are not immune to the internal dynamics which affect all groups. For example, groups will sometimes generate a particular viewpoint and members not subscribing to that viewpoint may be made to feel uncomfortable. Similarly, group members can sometimes feel under pressure to engage in activities that they might otherwise not wish to be involved in.

Two experiences of group healthcare

> I went to this healing group in the village, and though there were other disabled people there, I was the only one who had a pain problem. Everyone kept making these silly suggestions about what I should do and because there were things I didn't want to take part in, like talk about myself, I felt really left out. One day, it came to a head. I told them all that they didn't know what it was like to be in pain all the time and walked out. I didn't go back.
>
> I love it: there is such a wonderful warm, healing atmosphere, all this love and hope in the air. Everyone realy feels that they are doing something to get better, not just giving in. You really have to go and experience it to know what I mean.

DECIDING ON A PROGRAMME OF HEALTHCARE

It is unfortunate that so many decisions about healthcare are taken in a slapdash way. All too often people find themselves visiting a practitioner on a one-off basis because a friend suggested it, or because they saw a sign in a health food store or because they felt they ought to be doing something.

> I tried healing at one of those alternative festivals. Then I went to this Quaker meeting house in town. It didn't do much.

I went to the homoeopath twice and though it did help a bit, I certainly wasn't cured. I rang him up, it took ages to get through, and he told me that he really couldn't discuss details on the phone and suggested I come in for another appointment. I was furious that he expected me to pay more money so I never went back.

Every Saturday for a whole year, we drove for two hours to get to the practitioner. Paulita cried the whole way and it never helped in the slightest.

I've tried everything: I went to this acupuncturist way out in suburbs once, what a rip off, all those needles didn't cure me. I did have an appointment with an osseopathist but I hated all that bone cracking. My wife even brought back some homoeopathic pills from the chemist, but I didn't think much of them either.

It is clear that these people are not going about healthcare in an organized way. Some of the mistakes they are making include:

- 'Treatment Shopping': trying whatever's going without having any faith that it could help.
- Failing to make a positive and informed choice of a therapy.
- Not knowing how to assess progress: either not giving a therapy a fair chance to work before dropping it or failing to recognize that it was not helping.
- Giving no thought to what is really wanted from healthcare.
- Failing to find a convenient and suitable practitioner.
- Expecting help to come exclusively from outside, never wondering 'What could I do to improve things?'
- Seeing therapy as an irritating expense, having no commitment to spending money on health.
- Failing to integrate complementary therapies with other forms of healthcare.

One way in which you can avoid such mistakes is to develop a personal programme of healthcare. Here are some suggestions on how to do this.

1. Decide on what you want from healthcare

The fundamental question for anyone planning a programme of healthcare is: 'What do I really want and what am I hoping to achieve?' It is important to be specific and to think about particular problems and particular goals, both of which you should define as accurately as possible. By the way, you don't have to be constrained by conventional medical thinking on what constitutes a health problem. Though 'feeling a bit tired and irritable' is not a medical diagnosis, there is no reason why you should not consider its alleviation to be a goal of your healthcare programme.

Of course, one stumbling block might be whether your goals are realistic. It is tempting to set goals such as: 'I want to be totally pain free'; 'I want to wake up every morning full of vim and vigour' or 'I want to have a calm mind and relaxed body at all times'. It can never be overstated that complementary healthcare will not solve all your problems or make you feel 100% wonderful all the time. More specifically, there are certain health problems which might be beyond any complementary or indeed any other form of medicine (see page 43). Perhaps most important of all, it is better to set a number of small goals you can be fairly sure of attaining rather than one or two 'pots of gold'. Big promises and big goals are hard to achieve and you might be letting yourself in for a disappointment. This doesn't mean you have to rule out all hope of big achievements, it means that taking things one step at a time is normally the best way of getting where you want to go.

As well as specific health problems, it is important to think about anything else you might want from healthcare. It could be important for you to get out of the house and meet people; alternatively, you might want one-on-one contact with a practitioner. Do you long to lie down, switch off and have someone work on you? Or do you want to play a more active part in healthcare?

2. Work out which therapies could help you achieve your goals

Once you have some idea of what you want from healthcare, you can think about choosing a therapy or discipline. See which of the therapies could meet your needs and pick out any that you find particularly attractive or interesting; remember to consider conventional medicine, physiotherapy etc.

You will also have to think about whether you might need more than one complementary therapy. At the beginning of Chapter 5 there is a brief guide to which therapies might be the most useful for a variety of disabilities and common health problems.

3. Decide how to integrate different therapies, plus self-help, into a single programme of healthcare

The most difficult part comes in integrating the various therapies, plus self-help measures, you have chosen into a single programme of healthcare. Money is obviously an important factor and you will have to make a decision about how much you are willing and able to spend. In this respect, it can be a good idea to go back over what it is that you are hoping to achieve. How important are these goals to you? How much would you pay to achieve them? Information on the costs of complementary medicine and on possible sources of funding is included in the Appendix.

You will also have to consider how you can use different therapies to address your various health needs and how your programme might develop over time. Another issue is self-help. What lifestyle or diet changes could you make? How should you find out about these? Though this might all sound a little confusing at first, it is easier to understand if you read some of the examples given in the box on page 70.

Combining therapies

One of the most difficult parts of deciding on a programme of healthcare is knowing how to combine therapies. Each particular therapy has its own particular strengths and weaknesses and it is up to you to juggle these to your best advantage. For example, the advantage of pain-killing drugs is that they do get the job done, a couple of pills and you feel much better. Their weakness is that they may not affect the cause of the pain, that they may be addictive and that they can cause side-effects. Playing to the strengths of pain-killers might be to avoid habitual use and keep them in case things get really bad. A less sensible idea, and unfortunately all too common in practice, is to take them over long periods of time as the sole means of controlling pain.

Try also to make sure that the particular strengths of the therapies you choose lie in different areas. Part II should give you some idea of what each therapy is good at; avoid two therapies which achieve similar things. Osteopathy and chiropractic provide a good example of two therapies with similar methods, techniques and aims, But perhaps the same could be said of massage and shiatsu; shiatsu and reflexology; healing and massage; aromatherpy and herbal medicine, and, some might say, acupuncture and homoeopathy.

Examples of good combinations of therapies might include:

- Acupuncture, which can lead to improvements in physical functioning and mobility, and physiotherapy which can help ensure the flexibility and strength necessary for such improvements to be maintained.
- Osteopathy to help correct structural problems and improve mobility, followed by Alexander technique – because effective use of the body might prevent the recurrence of the structural problems – and occupational therapy, to ensure that wheelchairs, aids etc. are suitable.
- Massage, which involves a practitioner, and meditation, which is self-help.
- Homoeopathy to deal with the day-to-day problems such as pain and fatigue, steroids to help recovery from exacerbations and physiotherapy to maintain muscle strength.
- Shiatsu, for gentle relaxation and stimulation, with homoeopathy, to help overcome specific problems such as recurrent urinary tract infection.
- Meditation as part of a pain control programme which also includes appropriate medication, physiotherapy, counselling, biofeedback and acupuncture.
- Drug therapy to control a disease with massage or healing for mental and physical relaxation and a better quality of life.

Consider also how your needs may change over time.

Finally, avoid falling into the trap of 'the more, the merrier'. Some people end up trying about ten therapies, all at the same time or immediately following each other. For various reasons, this does not seem to be as effective as choosing two or three therapies and committing yourself to just those.

See also the section on 'Choosing a therapy' (page 56) and 'Complementary healthcare does not replace orthodox medicine' (page 87).

4. Find suitable practitioners

Your next task will be to locate practitioners and, perhaps, books and other resources. Think about the sort of things you might want from a practitioner following the section on 'Personal preference'.

5. Make a commitment to a fixed trial period

Once you have found a practitioner, you will have to decide whether you want some sort of preliminary interview or whether you want to start right away and try a few sessions. You should also make a commitment to a certain number of sessions before making an assessment of how you are doing. It is all too common for people to try just one session, complain that it didn't do anything and quit. Others get into the bad practice of taking things one session at a time, deciding to go for another appointment only if things seem to be working out after the previous one. This is distracting for the practitioner and gives you a financial interest in staying unwell: not a good message to give yourself.

It is a good idea to decide on, and even pay for, somewhere between three and six sessions before deciding whether to continue. Perhaps the only exceptions to this are counselling and massage: if you really don't like the practitioner or don't enjoy the massage, there is not much point in going back for more. Also note that there are some things which definitely should not happen in complementary healthcare (see page 241) and you should consider ceasing treatment immediately in such eventualities.

6. Arrange your first appointment

Generally speaking, the sooner you start treatment, the better. For example, in one study on acupuncture for stroke, it was found that treatment was significantly more effective if it started within three weeks of the occurrence of the stroke.

7. Think how you will assess your progress

This is something worth discussing with your practitioner.

To recap, you will need to take the following steps in order to decide on your personal programme of healthcare:

- Decide what you want from healthcare;
- Work out which therapies (both complementary and conventional) could help you achieve your goals;
- Choose which therapies you feel to be interesting or attractive, those that strike a chord with you;
- Decide how much money you are willing and able to spend on achieving your goals;
- Decide how to integrate different therapies, plus self-help, into a single programme of healthcare;
- Think about how you could use different therapies at different stages of your programme;
- Find suitable practitioners;
- Make a commitment to a fixed trial period;
- Think about how you will assess your progress and make decisions to change if need be.

Examples of healthcare programmes

The idea of a programme of healthcare is perhaps best understood by thinking about some examples.

Though Justin is in generally good health, he has osteoarthritis in his ankles, knees and hands. He decides his main goal is pain reduction as pain is his most disabling and distressing symptom. He is also worried about the amount of pain-killing drugs he is taking. A secondary priority might be relaxation as he finds his job very stressful.

Looking through the complementary therapies, he ends up making a choice between reflexology, osteopathy/chiropractic, shiatsu and acupuncture. He likes the sound of acupuncture and he knows that there are some scientific studies which show it can be effective for pain. He also feels that it is more powerful and direct than, for example, shiatsu.

If things work out with acupuncture, he resolves to consult his GP on how best to cut down his drug intake and the best pain-killer to keep by for occasional use. He also buys a self-help book on chronic pain which has advice on relaxation, exercise and psychologcial ways of defeating pain. In the long-term, he pencils in physiotherapy and/or the Alexander technique as a means of improving mobility.

He finds the name of two local practitioners from the Council for Acupuncture and he makes plans to call them to ask a few questions and see if either strikes him as suitable. He decides to try six sessions of acupuncture at first, but he decides that if after three sessions he realizes he doesn't like the practitioner he will look around for someone else.

Jane has cerebral palsy and is a wheelchair user. Apart from backache and recurrent urinary tract infection, she finds it hard to pinpoint specific health problems: she just feels achey and tired and tense and she finds she can't get comfortable in her wheelchair. Her goal is to feel generally better in herself. She also decides that, if things go well, she will look at ways of coping with the urinary infections and perhaps learn a self-help technique.

Jane decides that the following therapies could be appropriate: massage, shiatsu, reflexology, healing, osteopathy/chiropractic. In the end she chooses reflexology, partly because she likes the idea of pressure points and partly because she is unsure of her feelings about a full massage.

As there is no single register of reflexology, Jane decides to contact two or three of the reflexology organizations, find the names of her local practitioners, and call each to have a chat and see which one she thinks would be best. She decides to try three sessions, and if these work out, she will try another nine. Otherwise, she will either look for another practitioner or another therapy, depending on what it was she didn't like. She also decides to talk to an occupational therapist about her wheelchair and her backache. In the long-term she thinks about homoeopathy or perhaps herbal medicine for the urinary infections.

Abdullah, who uses a wheelchair as a result of a congenital abnormality, has no particular health problems at all. Though he is basically fit and well, he is interested in learning more about his body and calming his mind, which, he says, gets very cluttered after a day at work.

He likes the sound of yoga and meditation. He decides to start a meditation class right away and he starts looking for a yoga teacher appropriate for his needs. He also decides not to watch TV (unless there is a programme he knows he wants to watch) and to cut down his large intake of coffee and tea.

Chris was recently diagnosed with multiple sclerosis. Though his two most troublesome symptoms are currently fatigue and urinary urgency, he is primarily interested in preventing any worsening of his condition.

Having read about the importance of nutrition, Chris decides to go on the special multiple sclerosis diet immediately. He is confident of his ability to follow the diet, so he does not feel it would be of any benefit to contact a professional nutritionist. Chris also thinks about acupuncture, homoeopathy and reflexology. In the end he chooses homoeopathy, in part because his sister was succesfully treated for eczema by a local homoeopath. He decides to book a few sessions with his practitioner; however, he keeps an open mind. If things don't work out, he decides to try acupuncture. In addition, he leaves open the possibility of something like massage or healing, depending on how the money goes.

Chris also resolves to contact his GP about physiotherapy and exercise. In the medium term, Chris considers counselling: since the diagnosis, he feels that there have been a number of thoughts and issues bubbling 'just under the surface' and he thinks that talking these over with someone might prove worthwhile.

If all this seems a little daunting, remember that your GP, physio or occupational therapist might be able to offer you suitable advice.

Some authors think that it can be a good idea to write down what you want to do and how you are going to do it in the form of a contract with yourself. A typical written 'programme of action' might include:

- The goal you hope to achieve;
- What actions you are going to take to achieve that goal;
- When you are going to take them.

When you have written everything down – remember that it is important to be specific as possible – add 'I hereby agree to the above' and sign and date it, preferably with someone to witness it. It might sound a little silly, but it is said to work.

Getting started on a programme of healthcare

It is not uncommon for people to wait and suffer for considerable periods of time before they take action. There are a number of reasons why this occurs: becoming aware of these may help you to avoid a similar trap.

- Fear of becoming dependent on a practitioner or of losing self-reliance.
- Visiting a practitioner involves admitting that you have a problem: at some unconscious level, many people find it hard to accept fully that something is wrong and that they need help.
- 'Therapy fatigue': some people have tried so many different therapies, drugs and practitioners that they become sick of the whole business. This has been described as a 'conditioned hatred of healing'.
- Uncertainty can be frightening and all healthcare involves some uncertainty as to its outcome.
- One of the most difficult things about a health problem can be making the mental adjustments to the restrictions the problem emplaces. Having made these adjustments, it can be painful to be given new possibilities, something which brings the threat of having to make re-adjustments in the future. To put it another way: health problems can be psychologically exhausting, and change, even if in a positive direction, requires psychological energy.
- The thought of sitting alone in a room with a stranger, and perhaps having to answer personal questions, can be frightening.
- 'I don't want to raise false hopes.'
- Money: 'I am afraid of spending too much, I've got other financial priorities, I'm not sure I've got enough'.

Summary

Finding a reputable practitioner of complementary healthcare is a task made considerably easier by the existence of professional registers. These are administered by governing bodies in therapies where there is broad agreement on the standards and competence of practitioners. In therapies where there is no single firmly established register, it is necessary to check the competence of practitioners by using a set of simple questions. However, making decisions about complementary medicine is more than just a case of avoiding quacks. It is also about positive choices of what you really want from healthcare and a means of maximizing your chances of success. In this respect, personal preference plays a key role. It is important to choose a therapy you believe will be of benefit to you. You should also pay particular attention to your choice of practitioner: many authorities say that the relationship between practitioner and client is one of the most important factors in complementary healthcare. In deciding about complementary healthcare, it is also necessary to consider how best to combine different therapies, including orthodox medicine, so as to use each to best effect. A useful way of putting all these considerations together is to write your own personal programme of healthcare. This involves decisions, such as that concerning the therapies you feel could help you achieve your goals or the amount of money you are willing to spend, and actions, such as contacting a practitioner and making a commitment to a fixed trial period.

Part two

The therapies

5

Where to look for information

This part of the book is intended to give a rough and ready indication as to which therapies might be the most useful for specific disabilities or health problems. It is intended more as a general guide than as a definitive statement. Remember that your own personal choice of therapy and, in particular, of practitioner, is of prime importance and should be given more weight than the recommendations given below. It is suggested that you read about as many of the therapies as possible, taking the recommendations only as pointers.

It is worth stating that each of the complementary therapies can be profitably used across a wide range of client groups. This is partly because many of the benefits of complementary healthcare, for example, feelings of well-being, are 'non-specific', and are thus irrespective of particular symptoms or conditions (see page 40). Certain therapies, for example healing or counselling, have no specific indications and are not mentioned at all. Others, such as tai chi or massage, are so widely applicable that they alre only mentioned where especially suitable.

Note: The phrase 'therapies which calm and relax' refers, in this context, specifically to massage, aromatherapy, meditation, yoga, healing, metamorphic technique and polarity. To a lesser extent, it also refers to shiatsu and reflexology.

DISABILITIES

Remember to look under 'Common health problems of

disability below. If something you are looking for is not listed, try Appendix 1.

Amputation

For phantom limb pain, check under 'Chronic pain'. People who have had amputations may develop unusual patterns of muscle use (see Osteopathy). See also Alexander technique and Feldenkrais for learning how use the body effectively. Therapies which calm and relax may aid the reintegration of body image (see, for example, the story of Peter on page 91).

Arthritis

See under 'Rheumatic conditions'.

Cerebral injury

Cranial osteopathy (see Osteopathy) has proved helpful in many cases. See also under 'Stroke'.

Cerebral palsy

For children with cerebral palsy, see Appendix 1. For problems of muscle tone such as spasm, spasticity and athetosis, see Acupuncture, Shiatsu and Reflexology; see also Osteopathy. Stress and anxiety can increase muscle spasm, so see Therapies which calm and relax. See Alexander technique and Feldenkrais for learning effective use and functioning.

Chronic pain

See the boxed section on pain. Self-help is seen to be an important part of overcoming chronic pain – see Meditation, Relaxation and creative visualization and Yoga. Acupuncture is a well known to be a powerful technique for pain problems, see also shiatsu and reflexology. Alexander technique can prevent the bracing of muscles against pain, something which can of itself contribute to a pain problem. For muscle and joint pain, for example, backache, see osteopathy and chiropractic. Therapies which calm and relax can be effective for short-term pain relief.

Pain

Pain which lasts a long period of time (six months or more) is normally classed as 'chronic pain'. Many authorities say that there are a number of characteristics which are regularly found in people who have chronic pain. For example, there is often a constant search for a medical professional to 'fix the broken part'; depression is also common, as is inactivity and dependence on pain-killing drugs. Such behaviours may be a natural and understandable consequence of being in pain, but they can actually exacerbate a pain problem. As such, many workers stress the importance of self-help in chronic pain: treatment strategies move away from attempting to cure the condition and focus instead on improving the individual's ability to cope and live successfully with pain. The aim of treatment is often stated as 'to control pain rather than be controlled by it'.

It is important that therapies for pain mentioned in this book are not seen as just another 'cure', but as part of a wider programme of healthcare, one in which self-help plays a central role. For more information than can be given here, see any one of a number of excellent books about chronic pain (refer to the 'further reading' section).

Friedreich's ataxia

There are some anecdotal reports of benefit from homoeopathy leading to a reduction in the severity of symptoms, without affecting the course of the disease. See also acupuncture. Reading the sections about multiple sclerosis in the following chapters will give you an insight into the complementary treatment of disabling disease. See also the section on disabling disease in Chapter 2.

Huntington's chorea

The same applies as for 'Friedreich's ataxia'; see above .

Motor neurone disease

Some indication that acupuncture may lead to a reduction in the severity of symptoms without affecting the course of the disease. Similarly, practitioners of osteopathy and chiropractic have reported that they were able to improve quality of life in motor neurone disease. Reading about multiple sclerosis in Chapters 6 to 12 will give you an insight into the complementary treatment of disabling disease. See also the section on disabling disease in Chapter 2.

Multiple sclerosis (MS)

See the section on nutrition in Chapter 11 for a discussion of diet and MS. Self-help is an important part of managing any long-term disease: see Meditation, Relaxation and creative visualization and, especially, Yoga, which is very popular amongst people with MS. See homoeopathy and acupuncture for therapies to control disease progression. Reflexology is said to be useful for bladder problems such as urgency or incontinence; Alexander technique and Feldenkrais may aid rehabilitation; finally, practitioners of osteopathy and chiropractic say that adjustments to the skeleton can prevent bones impinging on nerves and therefore maximize the functioning of the nervous system.

Paget's disease

No reports of any effects on disease progression, but look under 'Chronic pain', above. Reading about multiple sclerosis in the following chapters will give you an insight into the complementary treatment of disabling disease. (See also the section on disabling disease in Chapter 2.)

Parkinson's disease

There have been anecdotal reports of the control of some symptoms through homoeopathy and herbal medicine. See also acupuncture. Some reports that meditation, relaxation and creative visualization and yoga have been of benefit in calming the body and controlling tremor. Reading about multiple sclerosis in the following chapters will give you an insight into the complementary treatment of disabling disease. (See also the section on disabling disease in Chapter 2.)

Polio

Some people who have had polio report that osteopathy, chiropractic and rolfing have helped with structural problems of the body. For effective mobility, see Alexander technique and Feldenkrais.

Rheumatic conditions

Check also under 'Chronic pain'. Complementary practitioners sometimes divide rheumatic conditions into two categories. 'Systemic' conditions are those in which symptoms commonly occur in parts of the body other than the joints; examples include rheumatoid arthritis (RA), fibrositis and lupus (SLE). These conditions (especially RA) respond well to homoeopathy and nutrition. See also Herbal medicine. In 'non-systemic' conditions, for example, osteoarthritis, symptoms are restricted primarily to joints and surrounding tissue. These conditions respond less dramatically to homoeopathy and the role of nutrition is less clear. However, acupuncture is effective for relieving pain and may affect disease progression. For all rheumatic conditions, osteopathy and chiropractic may ease stiff joints and muscles, leading to pain relief and increased mobility, but it can be unwise to use manipulation for damaged joints or during an acute attack. Yoga and tai chi can also help with mobility.

Spina bifida

For spina bifida cystica, see Alexander technique and Feldenkrais for improved physical mobility. For spina bifida occulta, some anecdotal reports indicate that osteopathy and chiropractic may aid incontinency problems. For better mobility, see Alexander technique and Feldenkrais.

Spinal cord injury

For phantom pain problems, look under 'Chronic pain' above. For improved mobility, see Alexander technique and Feldenkrais.

Stroke

There is some evidence that acupuncture may aid recovery of physical function after a stroke. For effective mobility, see Alexander technique and Feldenkrais. Therapies which calm and relax may aid the reintegration of body image.

COMMON HEALTH PROBLEMS OF DISABILITY

Aphasia

See acupuncture and osteopathy.

Back pain

See 'Chronic pain'. Osteopathy, chiropractic and Alexander technique are widely regarded to be useful therapies for back pain.

Bed sores

See 'Pressure sores'.

Bladder problems

See 'Urinary tract infections' and/or 'Incontinence'.

Bowel problems

Almost all complementary therapies seem particularly effective at addressing problems such as constipation and diarrhoea. In particular, see homoeopathy, herbal medicine, nutrition, acupuncture and reflexology. For irritable bowel syndrome (bowel pain with constipation or diarrhoea, not attributable to some other cause) see also hypnotherapy and meditation, relaxation and creative visualization.

Circulation

All therapies involving touch can improve circulation. For example, see Massage, Aromatherapy, Osteopathy, Reflexology and Shiatsu. See also Homoeopathy.

Constipation

See 'Bowel problems'.

Contracture

The prevention and treatment of contracture should best be left to physiotherapists and other conventional medical practitioners. However, any technique involving touch, for example, osteopathy or massage can be a useful additional therapy.

Cramps

See 'Muscle pain/cramps'.

Diarrhoea

See 'Bowel problems'

Digestion/appetite

It appears that almost all complementary therapies improve digestion and appetite. However, see in particular herbal medicine and nutrition.

Drug side-effects

Decreased need for drugs is commonly reported by those using complementary healthcare. The use of acupuncture and homoeopathy to treat drug side-effects and dependence is controversial.

Incontinence

See Acupuncture, Reflexology and Shiatsu. Some continence problems, for example, in spinal cord injuries, are unlikely to be susceptible to treatment.

Irritable bowel syndrome

See 'Bowel problems'.

Muscle pain/cramps

Almost all therapies can help muscle pain and cramps. See especially osteopathy, Alexander technique and homoeopathy. For self-help, see yoga and tai chi.

Oedema

Frequently helped by the therapies listed under 'Circulation', above.

Pain

See under 'Chronic pain', above.

Pressure sores

The prevention and treatment of pressure sores is best left to occupational therapists and other conventional medical practitioners. However, herbal and homoeopathic preparations can improve the rate of wound healing.

Respiratory infections/recurrent influenza

See homoeopathy, aromatherapy, acupuncture, reflexology and shiatsu.

Scoliosis

Some correction, and certainly a degree of pain relief, may be possible with osteopathy and chiropractic.

Sleep difficulties

Improved sleep is very commonly reported regardless of the therapy concerned. See in particular Therapies which relax and calm; for self-help, see Meditation, Relaxation and creative visualization. Homoeopathy, Herbal medicine and Nutrition may also be of benefit.

Spasm associated with neurological impairment

It is very difficult to make generalizations about spasm.

Therapies which relax and calm reputedly reduce spasm, though this does seem to be a short-term effect only. Osteopathy and chiropractic may help in certain cases. Spasm can sometimes be caused or maintained by the holding of muscle in tension so see Meditation, Relaxation and creative visualization and the Alexander technique and Feldenkrais.

Swelling

See under 'Oedema'.

Urinary tract infections

See Homoeopathy and Herbal medicine. There have been reports that aromatherapy may be of benefit.

Urinary urgency/incontinence

See under 'Incontinence'.

6

Touch therapies

MASSAGE

Introduction to massage

Massage is the common root of all touch therapies; it adds few complexities to the basic premise that to be touched in certain ways is beneficial to health.

There are, however, different emphases in different styles. Traditional Swedish massage centres very much on physical aspects. Practitioners of this style see massage as a good way of doing things which are healthful for the body, increasing the blood circulation, improving muscle tone, easing joints and working on knots in connective tissue. In addition, Swedish massage tends to be more structured than other styles. Practitioners tend, for example, to distinguish strongly between different types of strokes and they will use these in fairly set ways, given certain situations.

Swedish massage has been varied and adapted in the course of time. One recent innovation is to give the more spiritual aspects of massage – relaxation, calmness, wholeness – a more central role in therapy. Some practitioners have also incorporated elements of healing and shiatsu into their work.

One modern form of massage is called 'holistic massage' and practitioners say that they aim to treat the whole person, physical, emotional and spiritual. The massage itself is more nurturing and comforting than the Swedish style and pain is avoided. The choice of strokes is more a matter of the practitioner's judgement than of protocol and the same is true of the amount of attention given to each part of the body. The aim of the massage centres around enabling the client to feel whole, connected and alive, allowing the client to get in touch with his or her body, to listen to it and to accept it.

Massage is a well-known and popular technique It does, however, have one main problem. In the West, touch and nakedness have become strongly associated with sex and this makes some people feel very uncomfortable with the idea of paying for professional massage. This problem has been exacerbated by the fact that some advertisements for 'massage' are merely fronts for those offering sexual services. However, reputable massage practitioners have a good understanding of the therapeutic use of touch: in practice, many of the anxieties that some people have about feeling uncomfortable, or sexual, during a massage are quickly diffused by the strong, sure and directed touch of the practitioner.

Visiting a practitioner

Practitioners of massage work from warm, quiet rooms. Sessions normally start with a few questions about your health and a brief chat about the massage to come. This is a good opportunity for you to state your preferences for the form of the massage. You might prefer it to be energetic and invigorating for instance, or pehaps more calming and soothing. You might also wish to mention any areas you would like particular attention paid to, for example, a sore back or cold feet.

The practitioner will then leave the room to allow you to undress, though he or she will stay if you need help with this. Privacy is normally maintained by means of towels; nakedness is not compulsory however.

Most practitioners have their clients rest on a special couch for the massage. You will be asked to lie still, close your eyes and refrain from talking unless necessary (for example, if you feel pain or discomfort). The practitioner will use oil, often scented with plant extracts, to help his or her hands move over the surface of your skin. A full body massage can last anywhere between 45 minutes and an hour-and-a-half, after which the practitioner will often leave you to rest for a short while.

This is not a set form however: massage can consist of just a good back rub sitting up in a room with other people. Most practitioners are fairly adaptable and if removing clothes or using a massage table is something which would make you feel uncomfortable, or which would be physically difficult for you, there should be no inconvenience in arranging some suitable position to work in. Many practitioners are prepared to do outcalls and a session will often consist of a gentle kneading and rubbing through clothes.

Perhaps the best thing about massage is that it feels so wonderful. A large proportion of people who visit massage practitioners have no specific health problems: they go for relaxation and for the pure physical pleasure that a good massage can bring.

'I enjoy the massage, I look forward to it. It's bliss.'

Massage and physical disability

The physical benefits of massage are well known. They include improving blood circulation, aiding pain relief and easing tension, cramp and stiffness in the muscles. Massage techniques are often used by physiotherapists for these reasons.

Massage relieves all the pain and stiffness in my neck and shoulders. It also gets the circulation going a bit: my feet are now warm and there is more feeling there.

In addition to aiding comfort, these benefits can sometimes lead to improved mobility. Mina has used a wheelchair since a stroke, several years ago. One of her main problems is severe swelling in her calves and feet, caused by the combination of poor circulation and constant sitting.

When I first came for a massage, my leg felt like a sausage ready to burst! It was very painful. Massage has helped reduce the swelling and pain and now I am more mobile. I don't have to plan trips to the bathroom and kitchen any more, I can get up and walk pretty much whenever I need to.

Another client made this comment.

My hands are now much more supple. Before, I couldn't really do things like making tea or taking a bath without help. Now I can do more things for myself.

Sometimes, however, improvements in mobility are relatively short lived.

> I feel marvellous after a massage, really supple. I can turn my head right round. But by next morning I'm just as stiff as normal.

It is worth saying a little bit more about pain relief and massage. Massage often has very powerful effects on pain, though these are generally short-term.

> I can't believe the relief I get! But it normally lasts only half the week and by the time my next session comes around, I'm back where I started.

Massage is believed to be helpful in painful conditions for a number of different reasons. Pain problems are often exacerbated by the bracing of muscles against pain – for example, when a person clenches their teeth. Working to relax those muscles can often bring significant relief. Some workers have also pointed out that massage induces changes in the hormonal

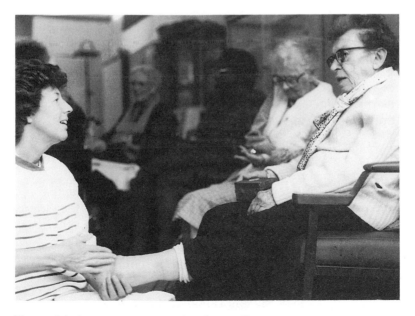

Figure 6.1 A massage group at a day centre.

and nervous system which would be of benefit in pain. For example, rubbing the skin is believed to release endorphins, a class of hormones which dampen down the perception of pain.

But it is not relief from pain that is most often remarked upon by people who have experienced massage, it is the deep relaxation that it can afford.

> The treatment is just so relaxing. It relieves all the tension in my back, neck and shoulders. I feel very calm and soothed afterwards.

> After massage, I fall into a deep, relaxing sleep. It's the best sleep I get.

Sometimes massage can bring about deeper and more permanent emotional changes. One practitioner described an experience with a client like this.

> At first, he was very tense, both in body and in mind. He used to chat nervously all the time. Now he is very much calmer: he almost falls asleep during the sessions and seems to have a much more positive attitude towards life in general.

Massage and body image

Body image and self-image are discussed in Chapter 2. There is little doubt that massage has powerful effects on the way in which people perceive themselves and their bodies and, in this respect, considerable attention has focused on the importance of touch. One practitioner put it like this.

> To be the recipient of a good massage is to receive care in the most direct and human way: through touch. It is to have someone say: you are worthwhile, I sympathize with you. A caring touch can communicate trust, empathy and respect. All this may be especially important for elderly or disabled people who may be rarely touched other than to be moved around.

It is interesting to compare this with the comments of a client.

> The massage makes me feel nurtured, cared for. It helps give me some of the emotional and psychological strength I need to deal with the multiple sclerosis.

The experiences of pleasure and well-being which massage gives can also play an important role. Simply feeling good can help people feel better about themselves in general: 'I feel more human after a massage' is not an untypical comment.

In her book *Multiple sclerosis: exploring sickness and health*, Elizabeth Forsythe relates her own experience of being massaged by a friend.

> My own angry feelings about myself and my intense dislike of my body made it almost impossible for me to let her near enough to touch me: I was frighteningly vulnerable. Her work ... began to lessen the loathing I felt for my body. It also relieved much of the spasm and tension.

A more complex issue is what a practitioner might describe as the 'integration of body image' or more simply 'body awareness'. Every person has a mental picture of their body and sometimes distortions or imprecisions in this picture can interfere with efficient functioning (see also the Alexander technique).

Peter was involved in a serious road traffic accident and despite extensive surgery and physiotherapy, he was left unable to stand for more than a few minutes or walk for more than few yards. A few years after the accident, Peter tried a body awareness course. He realized that the image he had of his body was perhaps as disabling as his physical limitations.

> I didn't want anything to do with my legs, I hated my legs, I felt completely separate from them. I felt my body was split in two.

Peter started receiving massage, and he feels that this put him 'back in touch' with the lower half of his body. Peter sees this as an essential step in his subsequent progress, believing that coming to feel his legs as part of himself once more enabled him to stand and walk more effectively. But Peter also says:

> The massage also helped me realize just how spiritually and emotionally needy I had become since the accident. These needs had been left totally neglected by all those years of surgery and physiotherapy.

Where disability has been caused by illness or injury, such as in the case of Peter or that of Elizabeth Forsythe, massage appears to be particularly effective at improving body image. Perhaps this is because, for these individuals, health and wellness is associated with a body they no longer possess. There may be the feeling that 'my body has let me down', or that 'my body is my enemy'. But those with congenital disabilities have also commented on improvements in body image and awareness after massage.

> When I was being massaged, it felt like a stroke up my back was traversing three countries. Massage made me aware of the splits and divisions in me. I certainly gain self-acceptance through touch.

Massage in practice

Finding a reputable practitioner of massage presents a number of problems. Firstly, there is no single, widely accepted register. Secondly, perhaps because of the nature of massage, the link between practitioners' qualifications and their ability is much weaker than in many other therapies. Thirdly, and worst of all, massage is sometimes used as a front for prostitution: most 'massage parlours' might more properly be described as brothels.

There are some registers, however, and these can provide a useful start. The London and Counties Society of Physiologists is one of the older and more traditional registering institutions. About 400 practitioners are listed as having skills in 'Body Massage', 'Remedial Massage' or 'Manipulative Therapy', depending on their skills and experience. The Massage Therapy Institute of Great Britain holds the names of about 600 practitioners, many of whom trained at the Clare Maxwell Hudson School (Clare Maxwell Hudson is a well known figure in British massage). The Association of Massage Practitioners is a much smaller organization and is based primarily in London: its practitioners tend towards a more holistic approach. Various schools of massage also keep records of qualified practitioners – the names and addresses are listed beow. It is also worth remembering that aromatherapists often use massage, so you might also like to try some of the contacts listed on page 97.

There is a massage division of the British Register of Complementary Practitioners and, given the confused nature of qualifications in the area, this might be seen as a useful resource. The register has two sections: 'Therapeutic Massage', for those with the ability to give a good all over body massage, and 'Remedial Massage', for those who have more advanced knowledge and who have the ability to treat specific conditions.

Finally, there are large numbers of massage practitioners who are not affiliated to any registering body. Good ways to locate such practitioners include personal recommendations and asking at natural health clinics and health stores. Be wary of massage which takes place in a 'health and beauty context' (for example, at a hairdressers). These practitioners often have little training. Also be wary of signs in newsagents and adverts in the Yellow Pages – it is rarely therapeutic massage which is on offer.

Many unregistered practitioners advertise as 'ITEC Qualified'. ITEC is a rather basic course which includes Swedish massage and elementary physiology and anatomy. Some people take ITEC as part of a longer and more thorough course, but there are those who take classes purely to get through the exam. It is particularly important to follow the advice on page 92 when trying to locate a massage practitioner. However, don't forget the central importance of personal preference. Try to have a brief chat with your practitioner on the phone first. It can be a good idea to ask about the style of massage practised (holistic? Swedish? vigorous? more soothing?) it can also be a good idea to try just one massage with a practitioner to see how you get on. If you don't enjoy it or feel better for it, it would probably be a good idea to look elsewhere.

Resources

London and Counties Society of Physiologists
330 Lytham Road, Blackpool FY4 1DW. Tel 0253 408443.

Massage Therapy Institute of Great Britain
Tel 081-208 1607.

Association of Massage Practitioners
Contact through The Dancing Dragon School, 115 Manor Road,
London N16 5PB. Tel 071-275 8002.

London School of Sports Massage
88 Cambridge Street, London SW1V 4QG. Tel 071-233 5962.

The British Register of Complementary Practitioners
PO Box 194, London SE16 1QZ (enclose a large SAE).

AROMATHERAPY

Introduction to Aromatherapy

Aromatherapists use oils distilled from plants for therapeutic
purposes. These 'essential oils', as they are called, contain a
concentrated mixture of the substances which give a plant its
own particular aroma; each is believed to have a variety of healing properties.

Most people are aware that our emotions can be affected
by smell. Many find that particular smells can provoke
childhood memories and it is well known that some odours
seem to be have fresh and invigorating qualities (e.g. lemon),
whilst others have a more warm and soothing effect (e.g.
sandalwood).

Aromatherapists use essential oils to stimulate or calm the
emotions, but they also believe that the oils have more specific
physical effects. There has actually been some sound scientific
research which supports the idea that essential oils can have
medically important properties. Some oils are said to possess
anti-inflammatory properties; others are thought to be
rubefacient (for blood circulation); carminative (for intestinal
gas); mucolytic (for excess mucus) and so on. Many of the oils
are anti-bacterial. In France, essential oils are sometimes
prescribed in place of antibiotics, especially for the control of
recurrent infections.

Essential oils can be used in a variety of different ways. One
of the most popular techniques is massage and in fact all
aromatherapists are trained in massage techniques. A few
drops of essential oil are added to the oil used for the massage.
The smell of the oils can add to its soothing, or invigorating,

effect. Moreover, the essential oils can be absorbed into the bloodstream through the skin.

Essential oils can also be used in baths, compresses and inhalations and various techniques can be used to vaporize oils so that their smell, and therapeutic effect, fills a whole room. They can be burnt in a special burner, placed on a special ring on a hot light bulb, or added to a bowl of hot water left near a radiator. On the continent, essential oils are sometimes taken by mouth, though this particular technique is prohibited in the UK.

Aromatherapy is one of the more popular complementary therapies, though it does suffer from lax standards of qualification and registration (see below). The use of aromatherapy in hospitals, special schools and other institutions is growing rapidly. Many people find aromatherapy's combination of massage and herbal medicine to be particularly attractive.

Visiting an aromatherapist

A visit to an aromatherapist will not be markedly different from a visit to a practitioner of massage (see page 87). However, an aromatherapist is likely to pay more attention to details of particular symptoms as these will affect the choice of essential oils. The practitioner may also give you some oils to smell so that you can choose some for yourself. You may also be given some oils to take home for use in the bath or a burner.

Aromatherapy and disability

Massage is an important part of aromatherapy, so you should read the section on massage in the early part of this chapter. Aromatherapists say that the use of essential oils increases their ability to bring about therapeutic change. For example, a person with arthritic pains might go for a massage to ease stiffness, pain and tension. An aromatherapist would be able to use essential oils to supplement massage techniques to bring these benefits: a calming and soothing oil could be used in combination with a pain-relieving oil together with one which is believed to improve the circulation. A combination of oils might also be given to the client to use in a hot compress at home. Some aromatherapists, however, may attempt to do

more than just relieve symptoms. For example, a practitioner
may attribute a rheumatic condition to 'a build-up of toxins'
and use de-toxifying oils accordingly.

Like massage, aromatherapy is deeply relaxing. Disabled
people who have visited aromatherapists have often found
benefit in the release of tension, increased sleep and so on.
But aromatherapy also seems to offer a number of other
benefits. Many people have found relief from various minor
symptoms after a course of aromatherapy. For example, one
woman who decided to try aromatherapy for relaxation (and
for the pure pleasure of it) found relief from troublesome
sinusitis. An aromatherapist who has worked with a number
of elderly and disabled people says that her clients often find
improvements in recurrent respiratory and urinary infections;
indeed, one French physician has found essential oils to be
a particularly effective remedy for recurrent urinary tract
infections and has reported on a successful case involving a
young boy who had a spinal cord injury. Aromatherapy has
also been reported to have been of benefit for skin conditions
such as acne and eczema, and for digestive problems such as
irritable bowel syndrome and weak appetite.

Aromatherapy in practice

Aromatherapy is one of the more poorly regulated complementary therapies. The training of some 'aromatherapists' consists
solely of a weekend course; beauticians, for example,
sometimes learn a few elementary techniques while training
in facials and leg waxing. The spread of essential oils into the
high street chemists will surely compromise standards even
further.

An additional complication is that many, otherwise fully
competent, massage practitioners may learn a bit of basic
aromatherapy and will occasionally mix together some nice
smelling oils when the mood takes them. Though this is
obviously somewhat different from the use of specific essential oils for a specific therapeutic purpose, it can sometimes
be difficult for members of the public to know exactly what
they are getting.

If you locate an aromatherapist through informal means,
such as a friend, or a sign in a health store, you should follow

the advice on 'How to check unregistered practitioners' given in Chapter 4. The resources list below gives the name and address of organizations through which you can contact a local aromatherapist. With the possible exception of the Register of Qualified Aromatherapists, the accreditation procedures used by these organizations may be far from watertight, so it may be worth following 'How to check unregistered practitioners' as a precaution.

Aromatherapy is generally more expensive than massage: essential oils can be very costly.

Resources

Send SAEs to the following.

Aromatherapy Organisations Council
3 Latymer Close, Braybrooke, Market Harborough, Leicestershire LE16 8LN. Tel 0455 615466

Register of Qualified Aromatherapists
52 Barrack Lane, Aldwick, Bognor Regis, West Sussex PO21 4DD. Tel 0243 262035.

International Society of Professional Aromatherapists
Hinckley and District Hospital and Health Centre, The Annex, Mount Road, Hinckley, Leicestershire LE10 1AG. Tel 0455 637987.

International Federation of Aromatherapists
4 Eastmearn Road, London SE21 8HA. Tel 081 846 8066

There is an aromatherapy division of the British Register of Complementary Practitioners, so you can also locate competent individuals through the Institute for Complementary Medicine (see page 276). Given the poor state of regulation in aromatherapy, this might be seen as a useful resource.

REFLEXOLOGY

Introduction to reflexology

Reflexology, or reflex zone therapy as it is sometimes known, is a special type of massage in which certain areas of the foot are seen to correspond to the organs or structures of the body.

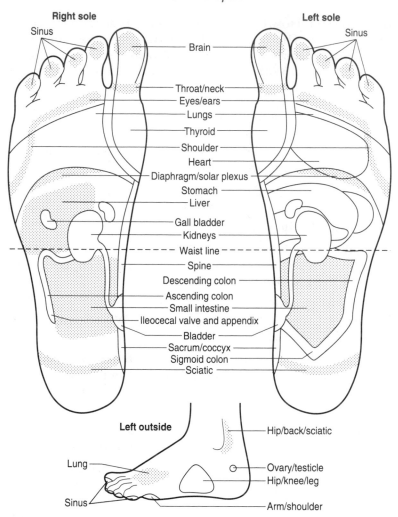

Figure 6.2 A diagram showing some of the reflex zones of the feet: these are thought to correspond to the organs and structures of the rest of the body.

By working on the feet, practitioners believe that they can stimulate healing in other parts of the body. Reflexologists see the feet as an anatomical map: damage or disease in an organ will be reflected in the corresponding area, or reflex zone, of the foot. By a careful massage of the appropriate reflex zone, the practitioner can help to remedy the disorder.

Reflexologists evaluate a person's state of health by careful observation of the feet. The bony structure, the colour and temperature, the condition of the skin and the tone of the muscles are all seen to give important information. Practitioners will also assess the state of each reflex zone by gentle use of the fingers. If the reflex zone is healthy, the only sensation which will be felt is pressure. If there is some disorder, however, a feeling of pain or pricking may be experienced. Such a disorder might be due merely to some immediate strain (such as will be felt in the eyes after a day working at a computer) but it can also indicate damage or disease, whether medically diagnosed or not.

Reflexology is probably the most popular complementary therapy amongst disability professionals such as physio-therapists and occupational therapists and it has been used successfully in a variety of rehabilitation settings. Though a treatment couch is useful, it is not strictly necessary, something which makes outcalls easy for practitioners and circumvents the need for transfers for wheelchair users.

Visiting a practitioner of reflexology

Reflexologists usually reserve the first appointment for a general case history and a thorough examination of the feet. Treatment normally starts with the second session: the prac-titioner will work on the reflex zones assessed as being disordered and attempt to bring them back towards a more normal state by a gentle set of massages.

Reflexology treatment is generally very relaxing and calm-ing. As the practitioner works on your feet, you will be asked whether you experience any painful sensations. The pain is not severe and feels quite unlike that which you might would get from an injury or joint problem. It may even be accom-panied by sense of well-being, somewhat like having a sore muscle massaged. You might find that you sweat during treat-ment, but you may also find that you feel shivery or cold, which is a sign of over-stimulation and you should tell your practitioner immediately.

If you have impaired sensation in your feet, you may not experience feelings of pressure or pain from a reflexology treatment. An accomplished practitioner should not find this a problem. After all, small babies and people in coma can be given reflexology. Interestingly enough, even if you do not experience much direct sensation from your feet, you will still find treatment relaxing, and you might also find yourself sweating or feeling shivery.

It is common for clients to experience diarrhoea, sweating or increased passage of urine in the first few days and weeks after starting reflexology. Practitioners put this down to increased activity of the elimination systems of the body and see such side-effects as a positive sign.

Reflexology and Physical Disability

Melanie Ryan is a Registered Nurse who has practised reflex zone therapy both in a private clinic and in a hospital setting. Many of what she sees as the benefits of treatment are among the classic non-specific, or generalized, effects of complementary healthcare (see page 10).

> I've done quite a bit of work with people who have had amputations. They all say that they get a great sense of well-being from reflex zone therapy and that they feel very relaxed after treatment. I always work on both sides of the body (sometimes I work on the hands) and the clients say that this makes them feel "equal" and balanced.

Melanie also uses a special technique called the 'sedation grip', in which the foot is gently held for five or ten minutes. She says that this can be very calming, physically as well as emotionally, for tremor can often be reduced.

Such benefits might be well predicted from the use of gentle and soothing touch. But practitioners of reflexology also claim that they are able to induce more specific improvements. One of the examples they give is the change in bowel and bladder function which so often results from reflexology treatment (see below). Many practitioners also say that mobility can be improved.

David has rheumatoid arthritis and is a wheelchair user. He made these comments after two months of weekly reflexology treatments.

> I feel stronger now, especially my legs: my walking is better and I've even driven a car a few times. I am much more confident in standing and my movements are less painful. I am much more flexible and my neck pain has eased. Perhaps best of all, my hands are now supple enough that I can do things for myself, like having a bath. I've learnt how to relax, both because the treatments are relaxing and through self-help breathing exercises. My steroid and aspirin intake have gone down. Every time I have reflexology I feel great, I feel I could get up and dance.

Sally Martin is a physiotherapist with long experience of reflex zone therapy. She says that in addition to pain relief and relaxation, the increased mobility and greater ease in moving experienced by David are very commonly reported by people with arthritic and rheumatic conditions. She says that reflex zone therapy can also help in stroke and multiple sclerosis rehabilitation, particularly as it can help reduce spasm and spasticity.

Erica, who has cerebral palsy, is one of those who says that reflexology has helped control spasm. This has made it easier for her to sleep and her speech has become much clearer. Her mother says that she finds her easier to handle in bed and that sitting has become less of a problem. But, as is so common, what Erica has noticed more than anything is that she feels so much more confident, stable and able to take charge of life. She was accepted by a residential school not long after completing the course of reflexology and she says, simply enough:

> Without the treatment I wouldn't have coped.

Reflexology and bowel and bladder problems

One of the most consistently reported benefits of reflexology is an improvement in bowel and bladder function. Whether it is a client relating their own personal experience of treatment, a practitioner discussing case histories or a doctor commenting on reflexology, increased continence and relief from irritable bowel syndrome are common topics.

Derek, who has multiple sclerosis, suffered from constipation and urinary urgency, which is when there is little time between realizing a need to urinate and absolutely having to go. He noticed an improvement in constipation after about four reflexology sessions and he realised that his urgency was decreasing a couple of weeks later. After about 25 reflexology treatments, his bowels were completely regular and the urgency much improved:

> I have much more control over my bladder. I can now always make it to the toilet, so I feel much more confident when I go out.

Reflexology in practice

The competence of practitioners of reflexology varies widely in the UK. At best there are physiotherapists with perhaps 10 years experience in a rehabilitation setting; at worst, there are those who learn a bit of reflexology on a weekend course and then set themselves up as 'Alternative Health Professionals'. Institutions professing to teach reflexology also vary in their methods and standards and there is a plurality of professional bodies, each generally associated with a single school and registering only graduates of that school. In short, the accreditation of reflexology practitioners is in a chaotic state and represents much of what is worst about complementary medicine.

On the plus side, the British School of Reflex Zone Therapy of the Feet (BSRZTF) is an excellent organization which has done much to ensure high standards of practice and promote the use of reflexology within orthodox medicine. The school only trains qualified health professionals, the majority of the intake being registered nurses, physiotherapists and occupational therapists. The disadvantage of the BSRZTF is that its members tend to have busy professional lives which restrict private practice and this can limit opportunities for new clients. Another useful resource is the reflexology division of the British Register of Complementary Practitioners, which is administered by the Institute for Complementary Medicine.

The Association of Reflexologists is one of the few organizations which was not set up for the sole purpose of accrediting graduates from an associated school. To be registered by the Association of Reflexologists, practitioners must have trained in an approved school, had one year's experience and provide examiners with a CV giving details of successful case histories. If the examiners consider the applicant to have a sufficiently 'professional attitude', they will be admitted to the register.

The British Reflexology Association registers individuals who have completed a course of study at the Bayley School of Reflexology. This is one of the oldest and most well-established schools, though there have been rumours that class sizes have increased with a corresponding drop in standards.

In conclusion, you have two choices if you are seeking a competent practitioner of reflexology. You can contact the BSRZTF or you can use one of the other organizations to locate a practitioner and then make sure for yourself that the person you are referred to is competent to practise. The section 'How to check unregistered practitioners' has information on some of the ways you can do this.

Resources

Send SAEs to the following.

British School of Reflex Zone Therapy of the Feet
87 Oakington Avenue, Wembley Park, London HA9 8HY.
Tel 081-908 2201.

Association of Reflexologists
27 Old Gloucester Street, London WC1 3XX. Tel 071-237 6523.

British Reflexology Association
Monks Orchard, Whitbourne, Hereford and Worcester WR6 5RB.
Tel 0886 21207.

British Register of Complementary Practitioners
PO BOX 194, London SE16 1QZ (enclose a large SAE).

HEALING

Introduction to healing

The most widespread conception of healing is that of a charismatic priest, an enraptured congregation and a fundamentalist, 'fire-and-brimstone' religious conviction. The goal of healing, in this view, is an instant miracle cure, a testament to the existence and power of God. Such ideas, however, do not accurately represent much of what is practised as healing in the UK today: the truth about most healing is much more ordinary, much less 'miraculous' and ultimately, perhaps, much more worthwhile.

The common belief of all healers is that a human being can induce healing solely by an effort of will. The details vary, but a common idea is that healing energy exists all around us and that the healer channels this energy to the person in need. This is often done through the hands, with the healer placing the palms of his or her hands on or near the person being healed. The majority of healers say that they can sense energy around a person and that where they place their hands depends on whether this energy is depleted or in excess in different parts of the body. Some healers try to assess and correct the energy at specific places which they call 'centres' or 'chakras'; others are more concerned with the state of energy in general. But it is important to remember that you do not have to share your healer's beliefs about healing, or about spirituality in general.

One of the advantages of healing is that it can be used in addition to any other therapy, conventional or otherwise. It is particularly worth looking at if you are unsure of what you want from complementary healthcare or if you are using therapies which do not concentrate on relaxation, for example, homoeopathy.

Visiting a healer

Healers work in a variety of contexts: at a client's home, at the practitioner's place of work, at a healing centre or even in a hospital. Some healers like to talk before healing, especially in the first session; others work entirely by intuition.

A healing session typically lasts between 15 minutes and an hour. The client usually sits upright in a chair, though healing can be done lying down. You will be asked to close your eyes and relax and the practitioner will place his or her hands in different positions on and near the surface of the skin. It is unnecessary to remove any clothes.

Healing is very soothing and calming but, at the same time, a feeling of invigoration is quite common after a session. You may feel a variety of sensations – heat, cool or tingling – and these can get quite intense. You might have a direct feeling of energy moving through your body. You will feel very focused during a good healing session.

It can take a little time to come back to reality after healing, so healers often suggest you lie down and rest for a while. Many healers use this time to talk as many people find it easier to communicate when they are calm and relaxed. Some healers lay great emphasis on the counselling element of healing. In the US, some professional nurses practise healing in a form known as 'therapeutic touch' and they often use the technique specifically to help patients put feelings into words. Some healers use the time after a session to advise changes to your diet and or to give you relaxation or visualization exercises to use at home (see page 147).

Healing and disability

One of the popular misconceptions of healing is that it is all about 'miracle cures'. From a disabled person's point of view, it is very unfortunate that this has become epitomized by the empty wheelchair or the no-longer-needed crutch held aloft: it distorts expectations, raises unrealistic hopes and involves a whole range of implicit assumptions that many disabled people find quite sickening.

Patricia, who has MS, gives a more down to earth picture of her experience of healing.

> I felt really, really good, really comfortable during healing, I felt a nice glow. The talking was important, it helped me get things in perspective, look on the positive side. Healing gave me hope!

Patricia does not talk much about her physical symptoms, though she did say that healing helped her knee when it was hurt in a fall. On the other hand Sam, who also has MS, feels that healing has quite definitely helped his mobility.

> You forget how bad you were. There were times when I couldn't walk or get out of bed. Now I can do things I couldn't do before, like getting on a bus or a train with a suitcase. Healing stimulated the 'I can do it!' feeling, I started seeing disability as a challenge. I had been trying to fight the disease before but I had no-one to help. Healing has transformed my life.

Others have noticed that pain and disability may still be present after healing but that their attitude to it has changed.

> The first thing I said to my healer was 'I've had five surgeries on that leg and I still have pain. I've given up.' But I did the healing and after the first session I cried a bit and I said all this stuff, it just sort of came up, that I thought that the amputation was a personal failure. Nowadays the pain is still there, but I can stand it okay.

Douglas, who is a wheelchair user said:

> I see now that there was no way that healing was going to cure me. But it did increase my mobility and it gave me peace.

His healer also noted that Douglas had a more positive attitude to life. Don Copland, of the National Federation of Spiritual Healers, says that such a change in attitude is one of the most common and important results of healing. He says that healing is a bit like using jump leads to start a car with a flat battery: one source of energy can be used to get another one going. In this analogy, the 'flat battery' might be seen as depression and negative attitudes, perhaps what you could call 'spiritual disharmony'. This can affect someone whether able-bodied, disabled, ill or medically healthy and not only is it distressing in itself, but it can cause ill-health or impede recovery.

Healers often describe their work in mystical terms. For example, one leaflet states:

Healing helps a person return to the wholeness of being. A wholeness which is his right in the plan of creation . . . The healer is striving to help the person find a balance again, an understanding. To do this he is used as a channel for the divine healing energies.

If you like to think of healing in spiritual terms, then you will have no problems with this language. If you do not like to think of healing in this way then it is worth remembering that 'spiritual disharmony', 'negative thoughts and feelings' and 'depression' are pretty much inter-changeable terms. And 'wholeness of being' could be re-described as 'feeling good, peaceful and positive about your life'. Whichever way you decide to look at it, healing can be very calming, very invigorating and has changed the way that many people look at themselves and the world about them.

Healing in practice

Healers are represented by various organizations. The National Federation of Spiritual Healers (NFSH) is the largest in the UK and it does not promote any particular religious viewpoint. The NFSH is a member of the Confederation of Healing Organizations, so its healers work to a strict code of ethics. The NFSH also provides an excellent contact and referral service and so there is no doubt that they should be the first point of contact for anyone interested in healing.

It is possible, of course, that you might have a particular reason to go elsewhere; for example, if you wanted a healer of a particular religious denomination. If you are unsure where to look, contact the Confederation of Healing Organizations.

You can also get healing in a group setting (see 'Group situations' in Chapter 4). Often a local group will take over a room or a hall for an evening and you can get healing there. Some of these places have a wonderful atmosphere and some people find it a more comfortable context than a one-to-one session. The down side is that you might not get to build up a relationship with a practitioner, that talking is difficult and that you might get only a short session of healing. Also, some of the centres are not wheelchair accessible. You can get details of healing centres from the NFSH.

Finally, if money is a problem it is worth knowing that many healers do not charge for their services, asking only for a donation of what you can afford.

Resources

National Federation of Spiritual Healers
Old Manor Farm Studio, Sunbury-on-Thames, Middx TW16 6RG.
Tel 0932 783164.
Send a request 'to be referred to a registered spiritual healer in my area' with a SAE.

Wilfred A Watts, Secretary
Confederation of Healing Organizations
25 Ducane Court, London SW17 7JQ.
Send SAE for details of other healing organizations.

There is a 'Healer Counsellor' division of :
The British Register of Complementary Practitioners
PO BOX 194, London SE16 1QZ.

METAMORPHIC TECHNIQUE AND POLARITY

Two therapies which show marked similarities to healing are the metamorphic technique and polarity. Each has its own particular world view and some ideas are particularly mystical. For example, metamorphic practitioners claim to be able to loosen influences which affected us before conception; polarity practitioners believe that 'energy flows via a positive outward movement from a neutral source, through a neutral field to some form of completion. It is then drawn back to the source by a negative, receptive pull'.

Like healing, both the metamorphic technique and polarity therapy involve ideas about energy. Blocks in the flow of this energy are seen to lead to ill-health or other difficulties; the therapeutic work consists in freeing up the energy, something which allows the body's self-healing systems to come into play. The techniques are not seen to provide specific cures for specific symptoms; the effects are envisaged in rather more general terms. Indeed, a metamorphic practitioner might consider a client's moving house (after a period of frustration and inactivity) to be an effect of the work.

The effects of polarity therapy and the metamorphic technique also appear similar to that of healing. Clients say that they find the treatments to be very calming, relaxing and restful. Many also notice that they feel invigorated, that their energy has been replenished. Some do notice improvements in mobility or in minor problems, but again, the most common theme seems to be: 'I still have my problem, but it doesn't trouble me so much'.

Ernie said this of his experience with metamorphic technique:

> It does work. It changes your attitude towards the problem, you deal with it and cope. It helps me psychologically, things don't bother or worry me, it is all just water off a duck's back.

Also in common with healing, these small-scale changes can bring great benefits for some people, the relaxation, calmness and increased motivation being just the right key to lead to significant improvements.

The metamorphic technique

In reflexology, the foot is seen as a physical map of the body, with specific areas of the body corresponding to various organs and body parts. In the metamorphic technique, the foot is seen as a time map of the body: a line drawn from the inside of the ankle along the arch of the foot to the big toe is seen to represent various stages during the time spent in the womb. Practitioners of metamorphic technique believe that our strengths and weaknesses are first fixed during this prenatal period. By working on the feet, they believe that they can loosen this 'time structure' and allow the life force of the client to be freed to alter characteristics formed in the past.

Practitioners of the metamorphic technique are absolutely firm about not treating specific symptoms. They use the analogy of a house: in most therapies, a practitioner will enter one of the rooms and give it a spring clean. In the metamorphic technique, all the doors and windows are opened and the fresh air is left to create balance and harmony throughout the building.

The practice of metamorphic techique involves a gentle massge up and down the insides of the feet and corresponding areas on the head and hands. The practitioner uses gentle, intuitive stroking motions and there may be some work just off the surface of the skin. It feels deeply relaxing.

Metamorphic technique is very easy to learn and it is common that, after a few visits to a practitioner, a family will be taught the technique to use with each other. This emphasis on self-help, and the awareness of the importance of family involvement, must be seen as one of the most positive aspects of the metamorphic technique.

The governing body of the metamorphic technique, The Metamorphic Association, seems to have a high degree of disability awareness. It has been particularly active in making the technique available at day centres, rehabilitation units and other institutions (where the response from the clients and staff has generally been very positive); and it has also fostered debate on work with people who have learning disabilities.

Polarity therapy

The philosophical underpinning of polarity therapy is that the universe is a manifestation of the interplay of positive and negative energies. Life is seen to be one particular movement of energies of these forces. Energy is seen to originate from a 'neutral source', become 'crystallized' in a solid form (for example, part of someone's body) and then return to the source. Illness is thought to occur when the solid forms are held on to and not allowed to complete their cycle.

Polarity therapists diagnose blocks in a person's energy system and release them by placing hands on the body in a systematic way. The energy is believed to flow between the therapist's hands so as to correct the imbalances. The physical contact in polarity therapy is much firmer than in healing or metamorphic technique and the practitioner may gently rock or caress the body or use light pressure on the abdomen to help ease the breathing. The originator of polarity therapy, Dr Randolph Stone, was originally an osteopath and naturopath and so both gentle manipulation and dietary advice also form part of polarity work.

Resources

For lists of practitioners, send SAEs to the following.

Metamorphic Association
67 Ritherdon Road, London SW17 8QE. Tel 081-672 5951.

British Polarity Council
5 Bullkamore Court, South Brent, Devon TQ10 9LQ.
    Tel 0364 42143.

7

Oriental medicine

ACUPUNCTURE

Introduction to acupuncture

Acupuncture is the best-known technique of traditional Chinese medicine, a system which also incorporates herbalism, massage, diet and exercise. The technique involves the insertion of extremely fine needles through the skin at special points; this is thought to balance the body's energy and stimulate healing.

The principles of traditional Chinese medicine are quite complex and can be difficult for a Westerner to grasp. The workings of the human body are seen to be controlled by a vital force or energy called *chi*, which circulates between the organs along set channels called meridians. There are 12 meridians, each of which corresponds to the major functions or organs of the body such as the lungs or bladder, and *chi* energy must flow in the correct strength and quality through each of these meridians for health to be maintained. Energy imbalances (which are associated with illness) can be corrected by a number of means; in acupuncture, needles are placed at special points on the meridians, and depending on how the needle is manipulated (for example, it may be gently twirled in place) the energy is either drawn to the meridian or dispersed from it. Herbs, diet and exercise can also be used to modify the energy state of the meridians.

Diagnosis in traditional Chinese medicine is very different from Western diagnosis. Whereas a conventional doctor will try to fit each patient into a particular disease category,

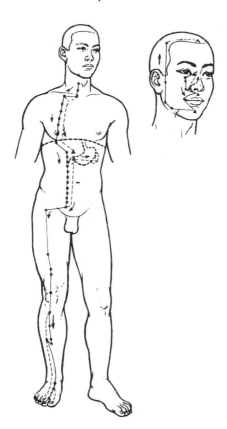

Figure 7.1 In acupuncture, needles are placed at special points along a channel, or meridian, through which energy is thought to flow.

acupuncturists attempt to assess each individual's particular state of energy. This is done by taking an extended case history, making observations of the colour and quality of the skin and tongue and by 'pulse diagnosis', a special technique whereby the energy of the meridians may be assessed by feeling the strength, rhythm and quality of the pulse.

Acupuncture is one of the most highly regarded complementary therapies. Large numbers of scientific studies have demonstrated its effectiveness and many doctors practise acupuncture either exclusively, or in addition to conventional medicine. Acupuncture is widely used in the pain clinics of hospitals and is seen by many to be an effective treatment for pain.

Visiting an acupuncturist

Most traditional acupuncture practitioners work from private practices with a comfortable place to sit and a treatment couch. In the first session, the practitioner takes a full case history, asking questions about lifestyle, diet, work and medical history. The tongue will be examined and a pulse diagnosis taken.

Needles will often not be used until the second session. On average, between two and six needles are inserted through the skin. They are left in place for about half an hour, and during this time they may be gently manipulated by the practitioner. Because the needles are very fine – not much thicker than a human hair – they do not cause pain in the same way as injections; in fact, it is possible to remain unaware that a needle has been inserted. If the needle is correctly placed at an acupuncture point, there is a slight feeling of heaviness or distention. Once they have overcome their initial nervousness, most people find that acupuncture is very relaxing and leaves them feeling quite 'up' and invigorated after treatment.

Practitioners of acupuncture also use a technique called 'moxibustion', which is the burning of a special herb (moxa) on, or just above, the surface of the skin. This is thought to have a warming and nourishing effect on the *chi* energy. Traditional Chinese herbal remedies may also be prescribed (see the section on herbal medicine in Chaper 11) and dietary advice is commonly given.

Some doctors and physiotherapists practise what is called 'Western' acupuncture. This retains the mechanical components of acupuncture (needles, acupuncture points etc.) but not its medical philosophy (*chi*, the five elements and so on). Western acupuncture might be offered by your GP or physiotherapist or in a conventional setting such as the pain clinic of a hospital. Its practice is somewhat different to that outlined above: for example, acupuncture points may be located using a special machine which measures the electrical resistance of the skin and diagnosis will take place along orthodox lines, rather than by using tongue and pulse diagnosis. See the section on 'Acupuncture in practice' (below) for more details.

Acupuncture treatment of physical disability

Acupuncture treatment of pain, disabling disease and stroke is covered in detail below. There are, however, a number of other common health problems of disabled people which can be treated by acupuncture.

Practitioners of acupuncture claim that they are able to strengthen the immune system and that this can help individuals overcome recurrent infections such as 'flu, or urinary tract infection. Acupuncture also appears to be a useful treatment for bowel problems such as constipation, diarrhoea and irritable bowel syndrome. Some practitioners say that they are able to control muscle spasm and spasticity in children but, other than the fact that any technique which involves relaxation can help spasm, there is not much known about this particular effect in adults.

Most people feel well in themselves after a course of acupuncture treatment and they may find that they have more energy in daily life. Improved sleep is also commonly reported.

Acupuncture treatment of pain

Acupuncture is widely regarded to be an effective treatment for pain. The fact that individuals can undergo major surgery without anaesthethic is a dramatic demonstration of its effectiveness. (It should be pointed out, however, that acupuncture for surgery is a particular and specialized use of acupuncture that you are unlikely to encounter on a visit to your local practitioner.)

Many people have found great relief from pain after a course of acupuncture. Some have discovered that pain was a large part of their disability and that its alleviation has improved their mobility and functioning.

Nathan has osteoarthritis in his hands, wrists and ankles. He visited an acupuncturist on the advice of his doctor.

> I was very cynical at first, I didn't want to know. But when
> the pain suddenly got extremely bad, I thought that it was
> worth a try. The pain is now much better: I have only had
> to take pain-killers four times last year. Though the stiffness
> is still there, my hands and fingers are much more mobile
> because, with hindsight, it was the pain which was stopping
> me doing things; for example, I never used to shake hands.
> My ankles hurt though, and I get stiff after inactivity.

Other people notice less specific effects on pain (see page 40;
see also the section on healing). Alan has a skeletal abnormality
which causes him pain in his joints and muscles. He tried
acupuncture when he became annoyed by the relative
inactivity of his doctor, who would only give him anti-
inflammatory drugs.

> Acupuncture changed my attitude towards the pain. Instead
> of feeling "Life is unfair, I hate this" etc. etc. I had a better
> feeling about my body and was happier to let things take
> their course. Though I am not free of pain, but what pain
> there is bothers me less.

Some people, however, find that pain relief is short lived.

> I felt great after acupuncture: full of energy and no pain
> at all. But by the end of the week I was back where I started
> and after a few months of this, I realised I was not making
> any permanent progress.

Another potential problem with acupuncture is that some
people with chronic pain regard it as just another 'cure'. A
number of workers have pointed out that in chronic pain,
'treatment shopping', the continual searching out of new
solutions, can actually contribute to a pain problem. It is
important to see acupuncture as part of a wider programme
of healthcare, one in which self-help plays a central role. (See
also the boxed section on chronic pain at the beginning of
Chapter 5).

Acupuncture and disabling disease

People with disabling diseases can benefit from acupuncture
in similar ways to other physically disabled people (and of

course, to the able-bodied too). Improvements in general well-being and the control of problems such as cystitis or poor sleep are commonly reported. But individuals with conditions such as rheumatoid arthritis or multiple sclerosis are also interested in the possibility that the disease process itself may be controlled by acupuncture treatment.

Acupuncture and rheumatic conditions

The scientific evidence makes it fairly clear that acupuncture can relieve pain in rheumatic and arthritic conditions. But practitioners claim that, in addition to pain relief, they are able to modify the actual disease process in rheumatic conditions: they say that stiffness and swelling can be reduced and that the progressive deterioration of joints can be reversed.

It is unfortunate that scientific studies have not investigated these claims, concentrating, as they have, on the question of pain relief. An exception is a Chinese study on lupus which did demonstrate significant benefit from acupuncture, though, of course, it is difficult to draw conclusions from a single trial. As a result, it remains unresolved whether acupuncture can alter the progression of rheumatic diseases such as rheumatoid arthritis or lupus. However, it may be worth drawing some parallels from the treatment of another disabling disease, multiple sclerosis.

Acupuncture and multiple sclerosis

People with MS commonly come to have negative attitudes towards themselves, their disease and treatment in general. Some have commented that such attitudes have been nurtured by the medical profession.

> When I was diagnosed, my doctor told me: 'There is nothing that can be done. Don't contact the MS Society and don't try HBO [a controversial medical treatment].' He didn't make a single encouraging or positive remark.

No reputable practitioner would claim that acupuncture can cure MS. But merely attempting to help and offering hope of some form of improvement can be enormously valuable.

It was good to have someone actually listen to me: just having the extra visiting time was tremendously important. My practitioner didn't make any promises, but she did say: "Let's have a go!" and that gave me a sort of hope.

One common result of acupuncture treatment in MS is the clearing up of minor symptoms such as backache or irritable bowel syndrome. Bladder problems can also be helped by acupuncture. This can be enormously helpful, not only because 'When you've got MS, you don't want anything else to deal with!' but because it demonstrates that improvements can be made.

There is little doubt that some people with MS do experience greater mobility and sensation after acupuncture treatment and that symptoms such as fatigue and urinary urgency can be controlled. Some cases have been especially dramatic, and though with MS it is always possible to say that these were spontaneous remissions which would have occurred anyway, the fact that acupuncture has received scientific validation for the treatment of pain makes it unlikely that 'spontaneous remission' would be an adequate explanation for all such cases. It would be true to say, however, that no-one knows how acupuncture affects the course of MS.

Dr Martin Allbright is a conventionally trained doctor who now practices traditional acupuncture full time. He says that the degree of improvement in MS is variable, but that it does depend largely on how much the client is willing to put into treatment. For example, unless a client exercises, any functional improvements made possible by acupuncture will be lost.

Dr Allbright also says, however, that the mainstay of his work with people with MS is 'gradually turning around negative attitudes towards treatment and disease'. It is interesting to compare this comment with a client's assessment of her treatment:

I feel I am getting much better. The fatigue is pretty much gone and I am back in work now. But the biggest change is that I feel I have a positive attitude, I am back taking part in life again.

See also the discussion of multiple sclerosis in the section on homoeopathy in Chapter 11.

Acupuncture and other disabling diseases

Acupuncture treatment of conditions such as motor neurone disease, Parkinson's disease and hereditary disorders appears to follow a similar pattern to the treatment of multiple sclerosis: a reduction in the severity of symptoms and an improvement in general physical and mental well-being. However, little is known about how the course of such diseases is affected by acupuncture.

Acupuncture and stroke

Practitioners of acupuncture claim that they are able to aid the recovery of sensation and physical functioning after a stroke. One of the reasons it is difficult to assess these claims is that people who have had strokes may gradually recover quite naturally. There have been a number of studies which seem to suggest that acupuncture is effective for stroke, but they are flawed by the lack of a control group (who do not receive acupuncture) to indicate how much improvement might have occurred without treatment.

Nonetheless, many people who have had strokes have found acupuncture to be beneficial. Jennifer's husband had a stroke and she says this of his progress with acupuncture:

> There is a psychological benefit, if nothing else. The physiotherapy has stopped and so has the speech therapy. At least our acupuncturist is doing something: the fact that he is making an effort helps my husband make an effort. His speech has definitely improved, and so have his muscles on the affected side, though there is still not much sensation, so he is pretty unco-ordinated. The main thing though is that I think he is more alert and aware. He hasn't had any depressions since the start of acupuncture treatment.

'Making an effort' is something mentioned by a number of practitioners.

> There is no way I can help a client without their active co-operation. They have to exercise otherwise any change that I am able to make will be lost.

The degree of recovery that is possible following a stroke depends on the severity of the stroke. Briefly, what happens after a stroke is that undamaged parts of the nervous system may take over the job of areas which have been destroyed. How completely this process is able to take place depends on the amount of damage that the stroke has caused. What practitioners of acupuncture say is that, given active participation of the client, and barring complications such as illness, acupuncture will help ensure the maximum recovery possible, whatever that might be.

Acupuncture in practice

The type of acupuncture described above is sometimes referred to as 'traditional' acupuncture. However, a number of orthodox physicians practise what is known as 'Western' acupuncture. Rather than assessing the energy state of meridians, the doctor makes an orthodox diagnosis and places needles in certain anatomical positions depending on the particular disease identified and, in some instances, the results of special measurements. The theory of Western acupuncture is rooted in standard anatomy and physiology: for example, researchers have linked acupuncture points to certain types of nerve endings and demonstrated that needling causes the release of natural pain-killing substances into the bloodstream.

Practitioners of traditional acupuncture say that because Western acupuncture forgoes the therapy's most basic theories and principles, it is not really acupuncture at all. Certainly the sort of acupuncture that GPs can learn on weekend courses might be seen to be a pale shadow of what can be achieved with this form of medicine, and some would doubt whether what is being practised is really complementary medicine or some strange variation of physiotherapy.

On the other hand, using a conventional doctor does confer certain advantages. For example, doctor acupuncturists have a great grasp of basic medicine and can call on a battery of diagnostic laboratory tests. This might mean that they spot something requiring immediate action which a non-medically qualified acupuncturist might miss. Though you can get around this problem by seeing your GP, practitioners of Western acupuncture also point out that their practices are based on firm scientific research, rather than tradition. For example, many of the scientific studies on acupuncture involved Western, rather than traditional practices. Finally, a relatively new form of acupuncture, laser acupuncture, is more widely practised by Western acupuncturists than by their traditional counterparts. In laser acupuncture, needles are replaced by a torch-like instrument which gives off a low-power laser beam when pressed against an acupuncture point. This method has several advantages: children are less frightened of the therapy, it is painless and it can be easier to use with people who have involuntary movements.

The section on 'Homoeopathy in practice' in Chapter 11 contains a full discussion of the pros and cons of conventionally trained and 'lay' practitioners of complementary medicine.

Resources

Details of your local traditional acupuncturist are available from:

The Council for Acupuncture
179 Gloucester Place, London NW1 6DX. Tel 071-724 5756.

This register also lists practitioners who also use Chinese Herbalism (see section on Herbal Medicine). If you are particularly interested in one or other of these forms of traditional Chinese medicine, you should state this when you contact the council.

Details of practitioners who have experience of work with children are kept by the:

Children's Acupuncture Register
City Health Centre, 36–37 Featherstone Street, London EC1Y 8QX.

If you do decide that you want to see a doctor, contact:

The British Medical Acupuncture Society
Newton House, Newton Lane, Lower Whitley, Warrington, Cheshire. Tel 0925 730727.

Finally, if you are frightened of needles, or if you think that using needles might be difficult (for example, if you have involuntary movements) a therapy called biomagnetics might be more appropriate: this involves the use of small magnets in place of needles. Remember that some doctors use lasers on the acupuncture points.

British Biomagnetic Association
The Williams Clinic, 3 St Mary's Church Road, Torquay.

SHIATSU

Introduction to shiatsu

Shiatsu is the one of the more widely established therapies which uses acupressure, the manipulation of acupuncture points with the fingers. Though there are a number of different forms of acupressure, few, if any, have developed the coherence of method and philosophy that is found in shiatsu.

Shiatsu developed earlier in this century in Japan, and its basic concepts borrow heavily from traditional Oriental medicine (see the section on Acupuncture). Health is seen to depend on the correct flow of *chi* energy through the body; ideas such as the meridians, the five elements and the pulses are also retained. However, there are several important differences between acupuncture and shiatsu. Firstly, because fingers replace needles as the primary means of affecting the flow of *chi*, the experience of shiatsu is more more personal than that of acupuncture, with the practitioner more intimately involved in treatment. Another difference is that whereas an acupuncturist will needle perhaps two or three locations during a session, a shiatsu practitioner will generally cover the whole body, though a few particular areas may be given special attention. Finally, an acupuncturist will generally attempt to make a precise diagnosis; a shiatsu practitioner is more likely to assess the 'feel' of a client and go along with that.

In general, just as acupuncture tends towards the more rational and exact, shiatsu tends the more intuitive and personal. In many ways, shiatsu may be regarded as a halfway house between massage and acupuncture. The use of touch, the involvement of the whole body and the more instinctive approach to diagnosis and treatment are important elements of massage; the concepts of meridians and *chi* and the use of special points on the body to bring about specific changes are principles found in acupuncture.

Visiting a practitioner

Unlike most complementary therapies, in which special treatment couches are used, shiatsu practitioners work with their clients on a thick mat on the floor. They also work through clothes: you should wear something light and preferably baggy to a shiatsu session. After a brief chat and case history, the practitioner will ask you to remove your shoes and any heavy outer clothing. You will then lie or sit down on the floor. The practitioner will start work fairly quickly: in shiatsu, diagnosis takes place during treatment.

If applied carefully, finger pressure on the tsubo (the shiatsu name for acupuncture points) should not be painful. There is feeling of heaviness and often one of well-being. Though these sensations are distinct, and though the practitioner may move your limbs and body during treatment, shiatsu treatment is generally very relaxing.

Shiatsu and physical disability

Shiatsu combines elements of both massage and acupuncture, so it is not surprising that the effects of shiatsu treatment include benefits associated with both of these therapies. In common with massage, shiatsu can ease muscular stiffness and tension, improve blood circulation and bring many of the benefits of human touch. In common with acupuncture, shiatsu is able to promote more specific changes in the body.

A particularly interesting shiatsu case history is that of Anton, who has cerebral palsy and is a wheelchair user. Anton has written this of his 18 months experience with shiatsu:

At the start of this year I was in so much pain in my body. I had pain in my back, my legs and my neck, but the worst pain was in my right side of my stomach. I was uncomfortable sitting in my wheelchair, I was sitting badly leaning over on one side. I was getting more and more tense in my body and I felt like my movements were getting out of my control, so much so that I felt as if I was going to fall out of my wheelchair sometimes. I felt generally unwell and I was losing all the confidence I had. I felt quite unhappy.

Since I have been having shiatsu, I feel so different in my body. I don't often get tense in my limbs and if I do, I know it will go away. I don't get pain in my left leg when I am using my computer now. I feel more solid in my wheelchair. I rarely get that terrible pain in my stomach.

I am eating very well, I feel stronger, I am sleeping good. I am happier, I still get my off-days but, as my parents said, most people get their off-days. I am relaxed and I feel great.

Anton's practitioner also noticed that though he normally had four or five colds a winter, he had only one in the entire period of his treatment. Anton noted that he now recovers more rapidly from the infections he does get.

Amongst other groups helped by shiatsu, are those individuals with arthritic pains. However, though pain relief tends to be longer lasting than that afforded by massage, it does not appear to be as dramatic as that provided by acupuncture. This appears to hold generally: in terms of specific and non-specific effects of treatment (see page 40), shiatsu appears to fall somewhere between the distinct effects of acupuncture and the more generalized benefits of massage.

It's certainly very soothing and relaxing: I almost fell asleep a couple of times. But there is also this feeling of balance, as if energy has been moved around. It's as if shiatsu goes somewhat deeper than massage, even if it doesn't feel quite so fantastic at the time.

Shiatsu in practice

The Shiatsu Society has an excellently controlled register, though not all competent practitioners are listed.

Shiatsu needs no special equipment and it is thus especially easy for practitioners to do outcalls.

Resources

The Shiatsu Society
5 Foxcote, Wokingham, Berkshire RG11 3PG. Tel 0734 730836.

8

Structural techniques

Many people are aware that osteopathy and chiropractic are similar therapies. In fact, the founder of chiropractic, Daniel D Palmer, originally trained with the founder of osteopathy, Andrew Taylor Still. In modern times, the two professions remain so comparable that a significant proportion of textbooks and journals are relevant to both. As the effects of osteopathic and chiropractic treatment are similar, they will be considered together. The term 'manipulative therapy' will be used to refer to both osteopathy and chiropractic.

Introduction to osteopathy

Osteopathy was founded in the 1870s by Andrew Taylor Still, an American physician who was frustrated with the ineffective medicine of the time. Still became interested in the importance of the structure and mechanics of the body and he formulated three principles upon which his new therapy, osteopathy, would be based:

- Structure governs function.
- The body makes its own medicines.
- The artery is king.

Contemporary osteopathy retains many of Still's ideas. 'Structure governs function' might be explained by using the analogy of a bicycle: if there are faults in the structure of a bicycle (for example, if the handlebars are not straight) the bicycle will not function properly: it will be difficult to ride.

Likewise, osteopaths say that abnormalities in the structure of the body, such as misalignments of bones, often lead to problems in the functioning of the body, for example, stiffness and pain.

Still's second principle, 'The body makes its own medicines' is common to all complementary therapies. Osteopaths see the body as having an inherent capacity for self-healing but they believe that this ability can be reduced by the presence of structural and mechanical faults. Osteopaths see their job as correcting these faults so that self-healing can resume.

Still's third principle, 'The artery is king', is retained in the assertion that the maintenance of a good blood supply to all parts of the body is of prime importance. Osteopaths supplement this principle with an idea from chiropractors: structural faults can interfere with the nerve supply. Much osteopathic work concentrates on the spine. The bones of the spine, called the vertebrae, not only support the body but carry a network of nerves and blood vessels. Faults in the structure of the spine (popularly thought of as a 'bone out of place') can distort or place pressure on blood vessels or nerve cells. This can cause pain and may also disturb the functioning of parts of the body and organs to which the nerves and blood vessels lead.

Osteopaths employ a variety of techniques to improve the physical structure and mechanics of the body. The best-known technique is called manipulation, or 'high velocity thrust'. This is when a practitioner uses a short, sharp manoeuvre to free up a joint, something which is often accompanied by a cracking sound. Practitioners also use more gentle techniques such as massage and stretching.

Osteopathy was originally formulated as a complete system of medicine but its emphasis has shifted in modern times. Osteopaths work with bones and muscles, so it is not surprising that they are most confident of treating bone and muscle problems. Most practitioners are wary of claiming that they can help other diseases – such as eczema or irritable bowel syndrome. However, many osteopaths will say that apparently unrelated symptoms do sometimes clear up after a successful treatment for back pain.

There are exemplary standards of training and registration in osteopathy and perhaps this is one of the reasons it is so highly regarded by the medical profession. Many GPs commonly refer patients with back problems to the local osteopath.

Cranial osteopathy

Cranial osteopathy, sometimes known as cranio-sacral therapy, concentrates primarily on the central nervous system. This extends from the cranium (the bones of the skull) to the sacrum (the flat bone at the base of the spine). Nerve tissue in the brain and spinal cord is attached to, and cushioned against, the bones of the cranium and spine by connective tissue known as meninges; circulating throughout the system is a special fluid called cerebrospinal fluid. Practitioners of cranial osteopathy place their hands on the cranium and sacrum of the client and feel for a rhythm which they say it is possible to detect. By working with this rhythm, and by gently handling the bones of the skull, cranial osteopaths say that they can balance disturbances and distortions in the nervous system.

There is considerable debate as to whether cranial osteopathy is a discipline in its own right, or whether it should be just part of every osteopath's work. It will be dealt with separately here on the grounds that its theory, method and experience are sufficiently different from standard osteopathy.

Introduction to chiropractic

An accurate description of chiropractic would not be very different to the description of osteopathy given above. The differences between the two therapies are primarily technical. Chiropractors believe that sections of the spine can become displaced and that these require manipulation to replace them; osteopaths say that this is rare and that it is much more often the case that vertebrae (the bones of the spine) lose mobility. Chiropractors pay detailed attention to the local mechanics of the spine. Osteopaths are more inclined to look at a person's overall posture and mobility. Chiropractors deliver a specific thrust designed to direct a vertebra back into position; osteopaths often use the limbs to make a levered thrust designed to improve the mobility of the vertebrae. Finally, chiropractors use X-rays as a routine method of diagnosis; osteopaths use X-rays far less frequently, primarily as a means of excluding disease.

It is hard to know how these differences might affect the client. Deciding between chiropractic and osteopathy is most likely to be a case of choosing the right practitioner, rather than the right technique, though you might particularly like the sound of cranial osteopathy or McTimoney chiropractic (see below).

Visiting a practitioner

At your first appointment, your osteopath or chiropractor will take a full case history, including details of your work, lifestyle and physical complaints. You will then be asked to undress down to your underwear: this allows the practitioner to observe the structure and movements of your bones and muscles more easily. The practitioner will ask you to make movements such as bending down or to one side so that your mobility can be assessed. Diagnosis is completed by the skilled use of the hands, though X-rays and other tests may occasionally be needed.

Treatment takes place on a low couch. Most of a session may be taken up with work on the soft tissues (the skin,

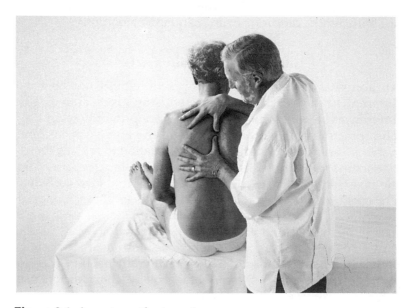

Figure 8.1 An osteopath at work.

muscles and connective tissue). As such, manipulative therapy is generally a very relaxing and pleasant experience. A high velocity thrust (when you hear bones cracking) is unlikely to be used more than once during a single treatment. The practitioner will explain what he or she is about to do and place you in position using pillows. The thrust itself is short and precise: it is an unusual feeling, but it is rarely painful or unpleasant.

Cranial osteopathy is a very different experience. It is very gentle and soothing. Some people say that they feel 'energy' being moved around, a little like healing. Others feel some form of emotional release:

> The first time, it really got to me. It felt like I was being all loosened up and released: I even cried a little.

Manipulative therapy and disability

Osteopaths and chiropractors say that physical disability often leads to unusual patterns of muscle and joint use; these can interfere with mobility and sometimes cause pain. Manipulative treatment aims to make structural adjustments to the body in an attempt to lessen these problems.

One case an osteopath used to illustrate this involved a 60-year-old woman who had mobility problems due to polio. The way in which she walked had led to excessive tension in some of her back muscles and to changes in the mobility of some of the bones in her spine. By using soft-tissue techniques to help ease tension, and manipulation to correct the spine, the osteopath helped the client's back pain and headaches and, to some extent, he was also able to improve her mobility.

Back pain is in fact the condition most commonly treated by practitioners of chiropractic and osteopathy. Stories where someone has crawled into the clinic doubled up in pain and walked out totally cured are not unusual:

> He turned my shoulders one way, my legs the other and then pushed down with his hands. There was a loud 'pop' and I suddenly realised that the pain had completely gone.

However, such cases are very much the exception rather than the rule, especially where back pain has been a long-term problem. Manipulative therapy is much more often a case of gradually improving the mobility of stiff and rigid tissues. Once normal movement is achieved, so say the practitioners, the body's own repair and maintenance systems can return to work.

Osteopaths and chiropractors like to emphasize, however, that they can improve mobility as well as deal with pain. One chiropractor worked on the rehabilitation of a young musician who was very badly injured in a car crash. She says that soft tissue and manipulative techniques helped to straighten the client's skeleton, an essential step towards recovery.

> With the hips twisted as they were, walking would have been just about impossible. I'm sure that straightening up the hips has been an important element in Don's progress.

Similarly, a practitioner who has worked with people with cerebral palsy has reported that a proportion of his clients have skeletal misalignments which exacerbate mobility problems. He described one client as having a 'tilted pelvis', correction of which made it easier for the client to walk.

Like many other forms of complementary healthcare, manipulative therapy also seems to bring a number of less specific benefits (see page 40). Jane is a wheelchair user who has been seeing a chiropractor for almost 30 years.

> A few things have got better, my bowel movements have certainly improved. But the main thing is that I feel great: it's like the work sets off a chemical in my brain which I can feel flowing through my body.

Manipulative therapy and rheumatic conditions

Manipulative treatment can provide considerable symptomatic benefit in rheumatic conditions by reducing stiffness and pain. Even the Arthritis and Rheumatism Council, who are extremely conservative on the issue of complementary therapies, accept that 'osteopathy can often be very helpful in the short-term'.

Pain from rheumatic conditions often comes not just from the joint itself, but from the muscles which surround the joint: these tend to be held in tension, as a sort of brace. Osteopaths and chiropractors say that soft tissue techniques such as stretching and massage can ease tight muscles and relieve some of the pain.

Manipulation of joints affected by rheumatic disease can also directly counteract stiffness and pain and thereby improve mobility. However, manipulation must be used carefully: it can actually be harmful if used on damaged joints or during the active stage of a disease like rheumatoid arthritis. Most practitioners are fully aware of when it is safe to manipulate and when it is not, but if this is something that worries you, do discuss the matter with your practitioner.

Manipulative therapy and neurological syndromes

Osteopaths and chiropractors say that they can help neurological syndromes such as stroke or multiple sclerosis in two distinct ways. Firstly, neurological syndromes very often lead to abnormalities of muscle tone, such as spasm or spasticity. Practitioners claim to be able to improve muscle tone so that such problems are reduced. Secondly, practitioners of manipulative therapy point out that if bones are misaligned, they may impinge on nerves, something which exacerbates impairment of movement or sensation. In the case of multiple sclerosis, for example, it is known that mechanical pressure on demyelinated nerves can provoke abnormal discharges. By ensuring that the bones of the spine are correctly aligned, osteopaths and chiropractors might be able to minimize such occurrences and consequently, reduce impairment. One practitioner has said:

> You rarely get to see a client long enough to assess changes in the progress of the disease. However, posture improves and you often do see some improvement in movement and sensation.

Cranial osteopathy treatment

One of the main uses of cranial osteopathy is in the treatment of children with special needs (see Appendix 1). However, cranial osteopaths do regularly treat adults: one of the most widely reported effects is a feeling of emotional release and relaxation, sometimes accompanied with an improvement in mental functioning, a sort of 'clearing of the mind'. Many people say they feel that they have more energy after cranial osteopathy.

Cranial osteopathy can also have effects on pain and functioning. Some pain conditions, for example, facial neuralgia, are associated with muscular and skeletal abnormalities in the head and neck region, the area of the body to which cranial osteopaths pay particular attention. The effects of cranial osteopathy appear to be most marked, however, for people who have suffered disabling injuries. Osteopaths say that trauma such as falls, head injuries or car crashes can cause displacements in the bones of the skull and distortions in the soft tissue of the nervous system. Symptoms which follow traumatic injury, for example pain or impaired functioning, are attributed, at least in part, to these structural changes. By using cranial osteopathy to correct such faults, osteopaths say that they can sometimes bring about marked improvements.

> The treatment decreased the sense of pressure and pain in my head and improved my mental function greatly from the level it had fallen to after the injury.

What are the differences between manipulative therapy, physiotherapy and massage?

Manipulative therapy differs from physiotherapy in a number of ways. Firstly, the treatment techniques used by physiotherapists tend to be different to those used by chiropractors and osteopaths. For example, physiotherapy treatments include exercise, surgical corsets and splints, traction, stretching and the use of machines such as diathermy (heat therapy) machines. Chiropractors and osteopaths depend primarily upon soft tissue techniques (such as massage and stretching) and manipulation.

However, manipulation is also sometimes offered in physiotherapy settings. There are technical differences between physiotherapy manipulation and osteopathic and chiropractic manipulation but the distinguishing factors from a client's point of view are less easy to explain. The complementary practitioners claim that they use manipulation as a part of a holistic treatment. For example, whereas a physiotherapist might treat a painful joint solely by paying attention to that joint, an osteopath or chiropractor is more likely to look at a client's work and general lifestyle and use the knowledge that stress can exacerbate pain problems. On the other hand, physiotherapists say that they have specialized knowledge of disability that manipulative therapists lack.

Perhaps the best way of summing up the differences between the manipulative therapies and physiotherapy is in terms of medical models. Physiotherapy uses the same medical model as orthodox doctors in order to diagnose and treat disease: chiropractors and osteopaths have developed their own systems. One of the consequences of this is that the relationship you have with an osteopath or chiropractor is more likely to approximate to the relationship you might have with other complementary practitioners. It is worth pointing out that a major study found chiropractic to be more effective for low back pain than outpatient physiotherapy treatment. However, many would argue that this was more a function of the pressure that physiotherapists work under in the NHS than any inherent differences in treatment.

The primary difference between the manipulative therapies and massage is that massage practitioners, unlike osteopaths and chiropractors, do not make an explicit diagnosis of structural misalignments. Massage practitioners may make some assessments as they go along, they might notice a particular part of the body being held tightly for example, but there is far less emphasis on identifying and remedying specific problems. Manipulative therapists do attempt to remedy specific faults and they may pay scant attention to areas of the body not required for this purpose. In sum, massage is a much more relaxing, comforting and nurturing experience: osteopathy and chiropractic are far more effective at bringing about precise changes in the body.

Osteopathy in practice

Osteopathy is probably the best-regulated of the complementary therapies. Training institutions are excellent and the governing body, the General Council and Register of Osteopaths (GCRO), runs an admirable referral service. Registered osteopaths use the letters MRO after their name. Osteopathic techniques are also used by naturopaths (see page 191).

The only thing you might have to worry about is if you particularly do or do not want to have cranial osteopathy.

Some practitioners use cranial work almost exclusively; others depend on it heavily; yet others use it only occasionally as appropriate. The best idea might be to telephone a few practitioners (always a good idea anyway) and ask exactly what their approach is and exactly how much cranial osteopathy they incorporate into their work.

Chiropractic in practice

There are two different types of chiropractic in the UK: McTimoney and standard. McTimoney chiropractors say that their method is more gentle and less invasive than standard practice. They point out that they rarely use X-rays and that their manipulative thrusts are specially designed to cause the minimum of pain and discomfort. McTimoney chiropractors also say that they always look at the whole body, rather than concentrating on specific sections of the spine. Regular chiropractors say that their standards of training and qualification are higher than in McTimoney chiropractic and that it is more effective to work on specific areas of the body than to try to cover the entire skeleton. Again it might be best to choose on the basis of the practitioner, rather than on the technique used.

Resources

The General Council and Register of Osteopaths
56 London Street, Reading, Berks RG1 4SQ.
  Tel 0734 576585/566260.

British College of Naturopathy and Osteopathy
6 Netherhall Gardens, London, NW3 5RR. Tel 071-435 6464.

For a McTimoney practitioner, send an SAE to:
The Institute of Pure Chiropractic
14 Park End Street, Oxford OX1 1HH. Tel 0865 246687.

For a regular chiropractor, send an SAE to:
British Chiropractic Association
29 Whitley Street, Reading RG2 0EG. Tel 0734 757557.
  If you include £1 in your sae, you will be sent a full register plus a variety of leaflets and other information.

Your GP might also be able to refer you to an appropriate local osteopath or chiropractor.

At the time of writing (1992), legislation is being prepared to pave the way for statutory regulation of the manipulative therapies. It is likely that this will improve standards of practice and consumer choice: however, some of these comments on practice and resources may become out of date.

ROLFING

Rolfing is named after its originator, Ida Rolf, though she herself preferred the title 'structural integration'. The aim of the technique is to align the body in an optimal position with respect to gravity, something which allows a person to stand erect, and make other movements, with less muscular effort.

The work itself consists of a cycle of ten sessions, each lasting an hour and each focusing on a different area of the body. Strong pressure is applied with the hands to parts of the body where muscle tendons are felt to adhere to each other, rather than sliding over one another in a normal way. As such, Rolfing is comparable to osteopathy and chiropractic except, whereas practitioners of the latter manipulate bones, Rolfers manipulate soft tissue. Another difference is that whereas osteopaths and chiropractors will seek to locate and remedy specific faults, Rolfers always work on the whole body: the ten-session cycle is used regardless of the client's state of well-being.

The pressure used in Rolfing is firm enough to cause pain, but this is often accompanied by a sense of well-being and emotional release. This is explained as follows: when we experience emotions such as anxiety, depression or fear we tense our muscles in characteristic ways. Sometimes, patterns of muscle use associated with emotions become habitual, almost as if the emotion has become 'locked in' to the body. Rolfers say that their work can help release these locked in emotions.

One Rolfer who has worked with a number of disabled people has found the technique more useful for structural problems than for neurological disorders such as multiple sclerosis or stroke. Some of the more successful cases he cites include severe scoliosis, polio and deformities of the lower limbs. He claims that rolfing improved mobility, eased pain and left clients feeling 'freer and lighter'.

Rolfing is a relatively new therapy. It is more predominant in the United States, where it is popular amongst physiotherapists and has even been the subject of scientific scrutiny. There are only a dozen or so practitioners in the UK, primarily in London and the South East.

You may also encounter 'Rosenwork' or 'Hellerwork'. Rosen and Heller studied with Rolf and developed therapies based on her work.

Resources

Rolf Institute
PO Box 1868, Boulder CO 80306-1868, USA. Tel (303) 449 5903.

The British contact for rolfers is Jenny Crewdson who can be reached on 071-834 1493.

9

Functional techniques

THE ALEXANDER TECHNIQUE

Introduction to the Alexander technique

The Alexander technique is named after its originator, F Matthias Alexander. Alexander was originally an actor, but his career was marred, and eventually ruined, because he repeatedly lost his voice. Alexander wondered whether his problem was caused by something he was doing, whether the way in which he was using his body was leading to the voice symptoms. By watching himself in the mirror, Alexander noticed that he was making curious movements with his head and neck as he spoke and by correcting these habits, Alexander was able to overcome his problem. This experience was the starting point for a number of years of experimentation, as a result of which Alexander developed the technique which bears his name.

The idea of 'use' is very important to Alexander teachers. All activities – sitting quietly, standing up, moving about – involve individuals in 'using' their body. One of the most important principles of the Alexander technique is that 'use affects functioning'; in other words, how we use ourselves in everyday life, how we sit, stand and move, affects the working of our bodies. If we use ourselves badly, our functioning will deteriorate and we may suffer headaches, back pain, or perhaps just a general lack of vitality. Correcting bad use may overcome such problems.

Traditionally, bad use is corrected by a vocal command of what to do. The slouching child is ordered to 'Sit up straight!'

Alexander teachers, however, do not instruct a person as to the correct posture for sitting, standing or moving, rather they are interested in the principles of good use. Simply speaking, movement should involve a lengthening and widening of the body and the absence of unnecessary muscle tension, particularly in the neck. Teachers of the Alexander technique are particularly interested in helping their pupils identify the habits which interfere with the body's natural functioning and co-ordination. Helping a person to recognize and 'inhibit' these habits is seen as one of the main purposes of an Alexander session.

As a method of learning, as opposed to a therapy, Alexander technique is not only used by people who have health problems. For example, many actors use Alexander to improve their body awareness. In fact RADA, the acting school, has employed an Alexander teacher for years. But Alexander can also be used as a healing technique: misuse of the body can cause or exacerbate pain and impede mobility; learning better use can help ease such problems. One especially attractive feature of Alexander is that it is, at heart, a self-help technique. One Alexander teacher, who has a disability, put it like this:

> Learning Alexander technique is like being given a tool: it is a very empowering experience.

Visiting an Alexander teacher

Alexander work is seen as the teaching of a technique and its principles, rather than as a therapy; hence the use of words such as 'teachers', 'pupils' and 'lessons'. The Alexander technique can be taught to groups, but individual lessons are more common. Simple activities such as lying down or getting out of a chair are used as a starting point: teachers give verbal directions, such as 'allow your head to ease gently up from your spine', and use their hands to guide pupils and bring their attention to particular parts of the body. In this way pupils come to recognize the habitual patterns whereby they have been misusing their body and, as an Alexander teacher might put it, be given the choice of a better use. A teacher may also hold part of the pupil's body as it moves and this can give the feeling of a fully supported movement, free of stiffness.

Contrary to what some people believe, Alexander teachers do not tell you what posture to adopt, or how to do a movement.

The benefits of Alexander technique are felt once a pupil incorporates its principles into everyday life. Learning how to sit, stand and move more efficiently will only bring improved performance, and relief from pain, if what is learnt is used outside the context of the lesson. This is another example of the way in which Alexander might be seen as more of a self-help technique than a therapy.

Alexander lessons often involve activities such as walking, climbing stairs, rising from a chair and sitting down. However, the Alexander technique can be taught to wheelchair users and others with more severe disabilities. Sitting and lying down constitute just as much a use of the body as more active exercises such as walking. In fact, Alexander teachers frequently have even able-bodied pupils lie on a table for part of the session. Alexander can also be taught by working with actions such as raising a cup to the lips or stirring a bowl, as well as with wheeling a wheelchair.

However, there are a few issues a person with a disability might usefully raise with an Alexander teacher. If you have problems with paralysis, or with spasm and other involuntary movements, it is worth remembering that an important element of Alexander work is the gaining of conscious control of the body. A teacher might therefore find it difficult to incorporate areas of the body, or movements, over which it is difficult to gain this conscious control. This is by no means an insurmountable problem, but it is certainly one which is easier to deal with by an initial discussion with your teacher. It is also worth pointing out that Alexander technique involves the belief that a person's functioning is primarily determined by the relationship between the head, neck and back. If you have impaired sensation or muscle strength, however, this may no longer be true. Again, something worth discussing with your teacher.

Alexander lessons can be intellectually tiring: it is hard work to pay careful attention to actions which were previously performed unconsciously. Moreover, the new ways you will learn of using yourself may not seem entirely natural, even though they may be more balanced and co-ordinated. It always feels strange to do something differently and sometimes this strangeness can translate into fear, especially if you are trying a movement or action you already have difficulties with.

But Alexander technique can also be relaxing. Sometimes you will be asked to sit or lie still and pay careful attention while the teacher gently moves and touches different parts of your body.

> I find Alexander technique very relaxing, sometimes I even fall asleep. The feeling lasts for the whole week.

Alexander technique and disability

Teachers of the Alexander technique often discuss what they call 'compensatory patterns' of use. To take a simple example, if someone gets a blister on one foot, they might slightly twist that foot as they step on it and place more weight on the opposite leg. This compensatory pattern can lead to problems

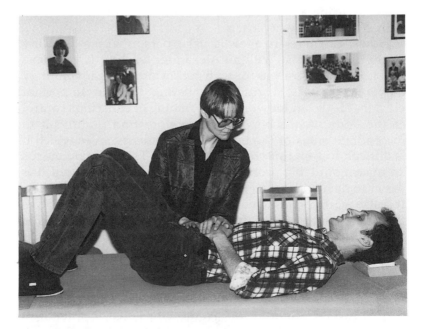

Figure 9.1 Part of an Alexander lesson may consist of 'table work'. Though the client looks entirely passive, the technique only becomes effective where its principles are incorporated into the client's everyday life.

of its own. It is clear that a disability can lead to all manner of compensatory patterns and that these might exacerbate pain and mobility difficulties. Alexander teachers say that they can help correct compensatory patterns which lead to such problems.

Martin has multiple sclerosis and experiences particular problems with his lower legs and feet. Martin's Alexander teacher helped him recognize that he was using a great deal of force, tension and pushing when he came to standing (a compensatory pattern). By using the Alexander technique, Martin was able to learn how to rise from a chair with somewhat less of a struggle. Not only did this result in his being less fearful of standing, but it meant that he endured less pain and tension during the rest of the day. Martin also says:

I think my control of my legs is now better and certainly my balance has improved. Sometimes I even suffer a sort of complete loss of balance and Alexander helps when this happens.

Such improvements in mobility are often reported by disabled people who learn the Alexander technique:

I used to get headaches from walking. But now I know how to use my body and I walk, and use my walking stick, in a more balanced manner.

I definitely find standing easier.

My walking and balance has improved.

Some Alexander teachers say that when people like Martin lose functioning as a result of disease or accident, they also experience a disturbance in the connection between mind and body. Simply put, the body doesn't do what the mind expects it to. Alexander teachers claim that they are able to help rebuild this connection. They point out that this is in fact the very aim of Alexander work, to allow people to become conscious of, to bring to mind, their use of their body.

An associated point is that because emotions may be held and expressed as patterns of muscle tension (see Rolfing) the releasing of muscles and opening out of posture that may result from Alexander work can sometimes also lead to emotional release.

When Rosie [who has a muscle wasting disease] came to me she was terribly fierce and angry. She was always talking about her pain and problems: she said that she didn't expect any improvement, that she hated her own appearance and so on. When she was nearing the end of the course of lessons she said she felt 'a sense of euphoria', that she was thinking more freely and that she felt more free in her body.

Alexander technique and pain

One of the interesting things about the Alexander technique is that, quite independently, Alexander teachers have developed ways of thinking about pain and muscle tension which are remarkably similar to those of orthodox practitioners specializing in the management of chronic pain. Both groups believe that the bracing of muscles against pain can itself contribute to a pain problem. Both groups also agree that chronic pain can often lead to a vicious circle: pain causes stress, stress causes muscles to be held in tension, tense muscles may go into spasm and spasm causes pain, something which kicks the whole cycle off once more.

Alexander teachers claim that their techniques may help to address these problems by bringing about a general reduction in muscular tension and by correcting compensatory patterns of use, where muscles are held tightly as a side-effect of a pain problem.

The Alexander technique can sometimes have powerful effects on pain. There are many reports of individuals who have overcome major pain problems as a result of using Alexander; moreover, in one study, the users of a hospital based pain management programme rated the technique the most beneficial of all the services offered.

But for people with chronic pain problems, perhaps what is most important about the Alexander technique is that it can combat the feelings of helplessness which so often result from long-term pain. The technique can sometimes offer explanations:

It's given me an idea of cause and effect. Sometimes I'd go for a few days without pain and when it came back I'd be all 'Why me?' With Alexander you realize it's what you've been doing with your body that often makes things worse.

Alexander technique can also offer practical help:

> Alexander technique hasn't cured me, but it is an extraordinarily good tool to deal with pain. I can now move without exacerbating the problem. Alexander also gives me a context: I see the pain as just one part of me, not my whole being.

In sum, the Alexander technique can increase the amount of control that people with chronic pain feel that they have over their health and their lives. This effect can have profound importance for those who feel that such control has been taken out of their hands by pain.

Alexander technique in practice

Natural health clinics and Adult Education centres sometimes run introductory classes in the Alexander technique. However, if you want to gain something more than a beginner's insight into Alexander, you will really need to contact the Society of Teachers of the Alexander Technique, who will refer you to a qualified teacher in your area.

Alexander technique generally involves more sessions than some of the other therapies listed in this book, perhaps 25 or 30 might be seen as some sort of foundation. This obviously has financial implications, though it is true to say that an Alexander lesson is usually less expensive than for example, an acupuncture treatment.

Alexander lessons can be given without the use of specialized equipment and, as such, many teachers are willing to do outcalls. To receive the most benefit from Alexander, it is necessary to incorporate what you learn in the lessons into everyday life. Alexander is not therapy, sessions with a teacher should be seen as a starting point.

Resources

Society of Teachers of the Alexander Technique
20 London House, 266 Fulham Road, London SW10 9EL.
  Tel 071-351 0828.

FELDENKRAIS

Feldenkrais is a technique whereby individuals can be taught to become more aware of their bodies and hence move and function more efficiently. As such, there are many parallels between Feldenkrais and the Alexander technique. Both methods work not with the structure of the body, as an osteopath would, but with its function. Alexander teachers talk about 'use' of the body; Feldenkrais workers focus on movement.

However, Alexander and Feldenkrais work in opposite directions. Alexander technique uses the mind to improve awareness of the body: it is a technique which depends on the ability to learn concepts. Feldenkrais work uses the body to 'program' (for want of a better word) the mind and nervous system and this process does not always require intellectual effort on the part of the client. So whereas Alexander teachers do not normally work with very young children or those with learning disabilities, Feldenkrais practitioners are able to work with a wide variety of groups, regardless of their ability to understand concepts.

Feldenkrais work incorporates two separate elements: Awareness Through Movement and Functional Integration. Awareness Through Movement takes the form of class practising special sets of small and unusual movements. For example, while sitting in a chair, a client might move one knee at a time gently forward while turning the head to one side, sometimes the same side as the knee, other times the opposite side.

Functional Integration is the hands-on part of Feldenkrais. The client lies passively on a low couch and the practitioner uses small, slow and gentle movements of the client's body. For example, a hard flat surface such as a book may be lightly pressed against the sole of the foot and tilted in various directions.

Feldenkrais practitioners believe that the body has an inherent ability to organize itself into movement. The aim of Awareness Through Movement and Functional Integration is to facilitate this process. Practitioners say that if the nervous system is allowed to experience various different forms of movement in subtle variations it will recognize for itself the most appropriate and efficient way of moving.

It is clear that Feldenkrais is very different from therapies such as Bobath (a type of physiotherapy) which attempt
to impose a developmental pattern and inhibit 'unhealthy'
reflexes. For example, Moshe Feldenkrais, the originator of the technique, once worked with a child with cerebral palsy whose legs had contracted together so that they
touched. Instead of trying to force the limbs apart, Feldenkrais gently pressed them even closer, almost as if he
was telling the nervous system: 'Look, this is how the
body is!' and allowing it to release the spasticity for itself.

Moshe Feldenkrais was particularly interested in the
problems of adults and children with damage to the nervous
system and this interest has remained amongst modern
practitioners. For example, a recent issue of the *Feldenkrais
Journal UK* was dedicated exclusively to this topic. There is
little doubt that Feldenkrais might have much to offer to
people with disabilities, particularly those with neurological
problems.

However, the work does have a drawback: its youth. The
first training for practitioners took place in the mid seventies
and the first British programme did not see its first graduates
until 1990. So it is likely that appropriate standards of training
and qualification are yet to be established firmly.

Other forms of bodywork

There are numerous different versions of techniques which,
like Feldenkrais, attempt to effect changes through touch and
movement. Practitioners tend to describe these as 'bodywork'.
Often they are offshoots of Alexander technique or dance
therapy and they frequently incorporate elements of special
physiotherapy methods such as Bobath or Conductive
Education. Practitioners tend to emphasize that their work
involves 'psychotherapy through the body' pointing out that
changes in posture and muscle tension often lead to emotional
release.

No doubt some of these practitioners are excellent and some
of their practices worthwhile. However, the need for caution
is indicated by the lack of registering bodies and institutions,

the disparate nature of the healing activities and the often unusual training of the practitioners.

Resources

Feldenkrais Guild
PO Box 370, London N10 3XA.

10

Movement and stillness: the disciplines

MEDITATION, RELAXATION AND CREATIVE VISUALIZATION

All cultures throughout the world have developed systems to calm and focus the mind and relax the body. Though meditation is normally seen as an Eastern practice, some types of Christian prayer might be seen as a form of meditation, as might rituals in which participants enter a trance.

Many of these practices have been developed for specific spiritual purposes. In the East, meditation is seen to calm the incessant chattering of the 'monkey-mind' and allow the recovery of 'intuitive awareness'; Christian meditation is about finding a greater knowledge of God. However, many people use meditations originally developed for spiritual purposes for non-spiritual ends: to achieve a peaceful mind, for example.

Meditation feels good: it is deeply relaxing and enjoyable. Some people say that they love the way that meditation allows them to 'sign out' from all the hassles and petty aggravations and take time to be with themselves. Others say that meditation calms them and helps clear their mind. But most people who meditate consistently will say that the effects of meditation spill out into their entire lives. The calmness and self-awareness become, after a while, not so much something you do, but something you are.

For some people, meditation starts as a spiritual journey, for others, it may become one. But meditation can be seen as something more practical and down-to-earth:

When I got to the hospital, a doctor started poking a needle in my eye to remove the grit. I became very still and calm. Later, the doctor said that he had never known anyone not to jerk their head back and move their eyes around while he was doing this. He also said that because I was so still, the whole operation had taken seconds rather than minutes.

I find I just don't get so infuriated and angry any more. When I feel a boiling point come on, I look at myself, and without any effort on my part, the bad feelings dissolve before my eyes.

Physical benefits of meditation

Proponents of meditation also believe that its practice leads to physical health and well-being. It is now possible to evaluate these claims because in the last few years, the effects of meditation on the body have been scientifically investigated. In a ground-breaking book called *The relaxation response*, Dr Herbert Benson reported on a number of experiments conducted on individuals sitting in meditation. What Benson found was that, no matter what the type of meditation involved, the physiological changes were similar. He hypothesized that all forms of meditation evoke a single physiological process and, in contradistinction to the well known 'fight-or-flight' response, he called this the 'relaxation response'.

The 'fight-or-flight' response is elicited when we are put in dangerous situations and it prepares us for physical activity. The heart and breathing rate increases, there is marked sweating and blood flow is directed to the limbs. Such changes were originally designed to enable us to run faster, or strike harder, and thereby escape predators.

The problem nowadays is that, though stressful situations continue to evoke the fight-or-flight response, we cannot respond by physical activity. Getting a tax demand, or getting stuck in traffic, cause the same hormones to surge through our body as does being chased by a hungry predator, but hitting someone, or running away is no longer possible. Some workers think that this explains why everyday stress can cause disease and they point out that the same hormones which are so useful in helping us to make a quick reaction in a dangerous situation may cause ill-effects if they continue to be released into our bloodstream, to no purpose, for years on end. For example, one of the changes caused by the fight-or-flight response is an increase in the secretion of certain acids in the gut and altered acid balance is thought to contribute to stomach ulcers, a well known health problem associated with long-term stress.

The relaxation response is seen as the opposite of the fight-or-flight response: each causes changes in the same bodily systems, but the changes occur in different directions. For example, when we are put in danger, our heart and breath rate increases, when we relax, our heart beat and breathing slow down. Eliciting the relaxation response by meditation or relaxation techniques can thus moderate the harmful effects of stress.

Different types of meditation

So far, the terms 'relaxation' and 'meditation' have been used somewhat loosely. Broadly speaking, 'meditation' normally refers to practices developed in the Orient and these place great emphasis on stilling the mind. Part of the meditation may involve focusing attention on the breath or on a 'mantra', a special word which is repeated over and over. Great importance is placed on allowing the mind to become empty of thought. A common practice is 'detached observation', awareness without judgement or expectation.

Meditation is practised with the spine in an upright position. Though some people who meditate use complicated positions such as the lotus, these are not necessary for meditation. The upright posture is necessary because though the body is completely relaxed, it remains poised and alert.

'Relaxation' is normally used to refer to techniques specially developed in the West to help individuals to relax in a concentrated and deliberate fashion. These techniques tend to focus on the body: many relaxation techniques involve a conscious effort to release muscle tension by slowly becoming aware of its presence. In theory, mental quietness and relaxation follow from this physical relaxation.

There are a number of different Western relaxation techniques. In progressive muscle relaxation (sometimes known as sequential muscle holding) different parts of the body are held very taut for a short period of time and then allowed to relax. This allows you to feel the difference between tense and relaxed muscles and it can also help you to learn about the areas of your body that you tend to hold in tension.

The premise of the Mitchell method is that characteristic postures are associated with stress. These include, for example, hunched shoulders and clenched fists. The method relies on consciously moving the body parts in the opposite direction to the tense position, so that shoulders are pulled towards the floor and fingers and thumbs are lengthened out.

Autogenic training is one of the more advanced forms of relaxation and must be taught by a trained practitioner, most of whom, incidentally, are qualified medical personnel. People who try autogenic training are taught to generate feelings of warmth and heaviness in their body, often by repeating phrases such as: 'My left leg is heavy, my left leg is warm, my left leg is letting go'.

In creative visualization, images are introduced into the meditation or relaxation. These might be of a general nature, for example, you might imagine a journey through a forest to a safe and happy place. But the images used can also be more directly related to health problems: cancer patients who use the Simonton technique might visualize their cancer cells as lumps of food being eaten by hungry fish representing the immune system; people with arthritis might use ripped fabric as an image to depict pain, and strong, mended fabric as the image to represent healing; some groups of disabled people might imagine energy flowing into impaired limbs. Another visualization exercise is to see yourself having solved a particular prolem: laughing and smiling, coping well, moving freely and growing stronger. Visualization is also an important element of hypnotherapy (see page 201) and of yoga (page 155).

Learning meditation

You can learn meditation either in a class or at home with a book or tape. Though meditation teachers are useful, and though a class can serve as a motivation and a focus for your meditation, it is not as vital to be taught meditation in person as it is to learn yoga or tai chi with an experienced practitioner.

It is important to use meditation and relaxation techniques every day, some say for at least 10 minutes, others think that two or three times that should be seen as a basic minimum. Meditation is essentially a self-help technique: individuals who merely go to meditation classes and who see meditation as something done to them rather than by them are not generally those who receive the greatest benefit.

Meditation and disability

For the most part, there is little reason why meditation should be a different experience for people with physical disabilities than for the able-bodied. There has been some discussion along the lines of 'Relaxation will help them deal with the frustrations of their lives' and plenty of patronizing asides such as: 'Autogenic training ... helps multiple sclerosis victims stay on an even keel'. It has also been suggested that meditation and relaxation training might prevent emotional frustration from interfering with rehabilitation. But the truth in these ideas only goes as far as the fact that meditation may help anyone cope with the irritations and hassles of their lives and prevent these from hindering the achievement of the tasks in hand. This applies no matter who you are and what you are trying to do.

However, there are three areas in which meditation and relaxation practices do seem to have special relevance for people with disabilities. The two most important are self-image and long-term pain; the third is spasm.

Self-image is discussed in Chapter 2. Briefly, many disabled people have problems with the image they have of their own body: they may see themselves as ugly or deformed, and, particularly, where disability has been caused by accident or disease, there may be the feeling that 'My body has let me down.'

In meditation, you learn to observe without judgement, to see how things are without forming opinions about them. Though this is a quite natural part of the meditation process, some practitioners have developed specific exercises to encourage such 'detached observation'. As an example, one of the exercises used by Barry Long is outlined in the box.

Meditation exercise

> Look at yourself in the mirror. See yourself as you are.
>
> *Watch yourself*
>
> Watch as thought tries to come between you and your reflection. The exercise is to observe your own reflection without making any mental comment.
>
> *Just see*

Ruth is a disabled person who started using Eastern meditation practices some years ago. She said that the first thing she liked about meditation was that it is 'self-directed', it is something you can do for yourself without the need for props or other people. Ruth also says this.

> Meditation put me in touch with myself. And I discovered that I was not my physical body, that I was not equal to, and bound by, this thing that other people called "deformed". Meditation became a relaxing and refreshing break.

After a time, Ruth's life changed so much that it took a 'skinny-dipping' party to remind her how far she had come.

> Someone made a comment something along the lines of how impressed they were that I'd joined in. I hadn't even thought about it.

Long-term pain can either cause or result from disability. The use of relaxation and meditation for pain problems follows quite naturally from the observation that pain, stress and tension can become linked in a vicious circle: pain causes stress and tension, and stress and tension make pain worse.

Nowadays, relaxation and meditation are a regular part of the work of many conventional pain clinics. One stimulus for this was a number of studies which showed just how effective meditation programmes can be for pain problems.

In one controlled study, 90 pain patients were given intensive teaching in meditation and asked to practice for 45 minutes a day, six days a week. Just over 70% experienced an improvement of at least a third; 57% achieved a halving or more of their pains scores. In addition, nearly three-quarters either reduced (44%) or eliminated (28%) their need for drugs.

However, perhaps the more fundamental reason for the growth of meditation and relaxation in pain work is the increased emphasis now placed on 'self-regulation', otherwise known as self-help. Medical practitioners who worked with people who had long-term pain problems began to realize that the conventional doctor-patient relationship – in which the patient passively looks to the doctor to cure him or her – itself contributes to the pain problem. This is because most people in long-term pain cannot ever be made 100% pain free. The real task, therefore, is coping with pain and making it more manageable – a task which can only be done by the individual with the problem.

It is interesting that most of the people who benefitted in the study discussed above commented that, though the pain was still there, their relationship to it had changed. For example, it didn't restrict their activities so much.

Spasm and spasticity can be made worse by anxiety and frustration. The reason that complementary therapies are reported to reduce spasm might well be related to their relaxing and calming effects. There has actually been a trial of relaxation for spasticity: a number of adults with cerebral palsy were taught progressive muscle relaxation and all showed functional improvements at the end of the study. If you have problems with spasm, you might see this as an additional reason to learn a relaxation or meditation technique.

Which sort of meditation or relaxation should I choose?

Relaxation techniques, such as progressive muscle relaxation or autogenic training are relatively easy to learn. Their effects are also very rapid and easily applicable in a wide variety of situations. Just try tensing up your shoulders or hands for 15 seconds and letting go, and see how relaxing that is. Many of the studies on pain have shown the effectiveness of the simple relaxation techniques.

Training the mind is much more difficult than training the body. Learning meditation takes much longer and is much more difficult than just picking up a few relaxation techniques. One estimate is that learning meditation takes about as long as learning a foreign language. The advantage of meditation is that it goes much deeper: people who meditate regularly say that it changes their lives and the way they see themselves. Others say that meditation can give meaning to what they do.

Finally, it is, of course, possible to learn both. Many people start with something like sequential muscle holding or a simple deep breathing exercise and graduate on to meditation.

Resources

You can find relaxation and meditation classes advertised in various places: health journals, newspapers, magazines and health shops. Most local councils run appropriate classes through Adult Education. Your GP might also be able to help you. You can find books on meditation and relaxation in both general and specialized bookshops.

Remember that there are many different types of meditation and relaxation, so if you don't like the sound of a particular class or book you need not think that meditation isn't for you. For example, some people have dipped into meditation books, found them full of stuff about Krishna and the various stages of heaven and abandoned the whole project there and then. There are plenty of more down to earth interpretations of meditation, if that is what you are looking for.

Further information is available from the following organizations.

Relaxation for Living
Dunesk, Burwood Park Road, Walton on Thames,
    Surrey KY12 5LH.

Autogenic training
101 Harley Street, London W1N 1DF.

See also the resources sections for yoga and hypnotherapy.

YOGA AND TAI CHI

Yoga and tai chi are not therapies, something done to you by a practitioner, but disciplines, something you can practise for yourself. Though each does bring a number of physical benefits, such as increased strength and suppleness, people who practise yoga and tai chi say that the benefits go far beyond mere changes to the body. Many people find that yoga and tai chi lead to mental and emotional calmness. At first, this occurs perhaps during and just after a session, but after a while, this calmness may be experienced throughout the day. Many people also feel that the practice of yoga and tai chi helps put them in touch with themselves, both physically and mentally: they may experience increased awareness of their body, how it is and how it moves, and they may come to a better understanding of their mind and emotions.

Many individuals also find that, as 'self-directed' activities, yoga and tai chi can be very empowering and liberating.

It is a way of doing something positive for myself, and I don't have to depend on other people or props of any kind.

Though much physiotherapy also involves self-directed activity, there are a number of differences between yoga and tai chi and the exercises you might be given by a physiotherapist. Firstly, yoga and tai chi feel good: tai chi has been described as a form of gentle self-massage and many people say that they feel relaxed and peaceful after their morning yoga session. Secondly, whereas physiotherapy exercises generally involve a degree of pushing and force and struggle, yoga and tai chi consist of more flowing, gentle and graceful movements. Some people prefer the more vigorous exercises, they like the sense of battling and conquering, of putting positive effort into a problem. Others prefer the more gentle approach, pointing out that it is often force and struggle that is preventing them from moving easily.

Another difference is that some people feel that physiotherapy exercises involve a sort of opposition between themselves and their body: 'My body is weak, I will work and exercise it to make it work for me'. Yoga and tai chi involve being with the body, not fighting against it.

An interesting expression of this can be found in language. A physiotherapist might tell a client to stretch such-and-such a muscle to ease spasm, to rotate a certain joint to prevent contracture and to work a particular limb to prevent muscular atrophy. A yoga or tai chi teacher is more likely to encourage a client to observe how their muscles relax and their breathing quietens, or to feel their 'centre' and the flow of energy through their body.

This might be an especially important consideration for people who have disabling diseases. Such individuals often feel that their body has 'let them down', that their body is their enemy, and some have commented that they would like this perception to be negated, rather than reinforced, by the exercises they choose to do. An associated point is that yoga and tai chi involve looking at diet and lifestyle (see below); some people see this as a much needed 'whole person' approach which differs radically from physiotherapy's focus on bones and nerves and muscles.

The final difference between yoga or tai chi exercises, and those of physiotherapy, is that the latter have been specially designed to help specific health problems and the fact that they are able to do so has normally been demonstrated scientifically. For example, a certain muscle stretch may have been found to ease spasm in certain ways: this will be prescribed to clients on appropriate criteria and one can be pretty sure that it will be effective. Many workers believe that the specific therapeutic interventions of physiotherapy and the more general approach of yoga and tai chi complement each other perfectly.

Introduction to yoga

Yoga is a system of exercises for the mind and body which is based upon traditional Indian beliefs about health. **Asanas** are the special postures which are the most well known feature of yoga. These vary in difficulty and complexity and there are postures suitable for all levels of ability and disability. Yoga practitioners believe that the asanas consist of somewhat more than just good stretches and exercises: asanas are thought to release and tone muscles and joints, massage the internal organs and promote better breathing and circulation.

Moreover, the asanas are designed to improve the flow of **prana**, or vital energy, through the body. **Pranayama** consists of a special set of breathing exercises, with particular attention paid to the proper and balanced use of the different sets of muscles used in breathing. Optimal breathing is thought to calm the mind and harmonize the flow of prana. Meditation is also a central part of yoga (see the section above on Meditation, relaxation and creative visualization): yoga meditation is sometimes known as **samyama**.

Asanas, pranayama and meditation are used every day, perhaps a half-hour session in the morning or before the evening meal. Some people find the mere discipline of practising yoga to be enormously beneficial. However, yoga can be taken somewhat further than daily exercises; in fact, many people see yoga as a philosophy, as a way of life in which the practice of postures and breathing exercises form but one element.

The overall aim of the yoga way of living is a calm and well-ordered life. Yogis (masters of yoga) believe that one's surroundings and dress should be kept pleasant, clean and simple: excesses and self-indulgence in food, sex and material possessions should be avoided, as should violence and untruth.

Diet is seen of prime importance in yoga, the emphasis being on the consumption of foods which increase vitality, energy and clear thought. Foods which lead to lethargy and dependence – such as coffee, alcohol and processed foods – are avoided, as are those which stimulate the body, such as spicy or pungent foods. Yogis also emphasize the importance of how you eat: meals should be taken slowly in a quiet and pleasant environment; stress and distractions should be avoided.

Yoga also involves examining the emotions: various techniques of introspection are used to diffuse negative emotions and to develop positive states of mind. The yoga way of life involves cultivating tolerance, understanding, love and compassion.

Yoga is perhaps the best-known and accepted form of healthcare covered by this book: it is extremely popular across a wide spectrum of different individuals. Though not everyone who practises yoga adheres to all of the wider principles outlined above, some people find the more spiritual aspects of yoga to be particularly appealing, something with which to make a new start in life. For example, a doctor made this comment about a middle-aged woman who contracted rheumatoid arthritis:

> She felt that if she could change herself, her disease would have to change too. Yoga provided the key to that change.

Introduction to tai chi

Tai chi is a gentle movement exercise which originated in China many thousands of years ago. It can be practised alone, in what is known as solo form, or in pairs, in 'pushing hands'. The solo form consists of a series of slow and graceful movements which follow a set pattern. This pattern, known as 'the form', is extremely precise and must be learnt and refined with a tai chi teacher. Pushing hands is an exercise practised in pairs: it develops the ability to push and yield by using sensitivity and balance, rather than brute force. Some teachers also teach **chi kung**, breathing exercises in which the breath is co-ordinated with simple movements.

Tai chi is based on Taoist philosophy. This teaches that the world is a manifestation of the interplay of two forces, yin and yang, and that life can be lived most effectively and happily if a person refrains from interfering with the natural ebb and flow of these forces. The movements in tai chi reflect Taoist beliefs: each move is seen to be created naturally by its predecessor so that no effort is required to enact the complete form.

Tai chi has been described as a 'non-violent martial art': simply put, the balance, strength and concentration which tai chi develops are used for health and well-being, rather than for violent ends. There are no 'belts' in tai chi as there are in judo and karate because tai chi is seen as an end in itself, something for joy and pleasure and personal development. (It is worth pointing out, however, that 'pushing hands' can be practised competitively: you should be aware that some teachers place significant emphasis on aggression and self-defence.)

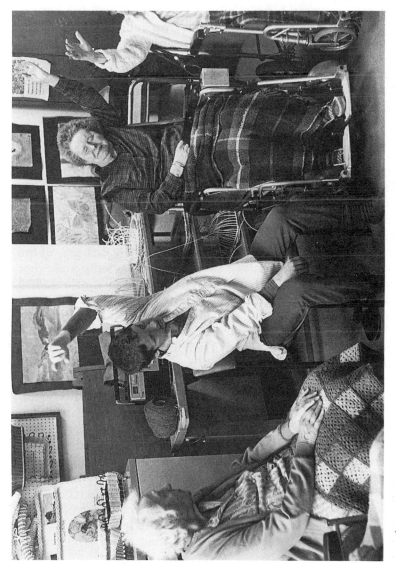

Figure 10.1 Tai chi 'on wheels'.

Though tai chi normally requires a standing posture, it can be adapted for wheelchair users. One of Britain's leading teachers, Linda Chase Broda, has developed 'tai chi on wheels', a special form of sitting tai chi in which the bottom replaces the legs and feet as the point for centring the distribution of weight and energy. Broda points out that the heart of tai chi is not the individual movements of the classical forms, but the principles upon which the movements are based, and that at least some of these principles are applicable, and valuable, for people who use wheelchairs.

Yoga, tai chi and disability

Yoga and tai chi are traditional elements of rehabilitation in Asia: Iyengar, after whom one particular form of yoga is named, became well known in India for his work with disabled people. In China, acupuncturists often refer clients to a tai chi teacher at the conclusion of treatment. In the West, there is growing recognition that yoga and tai chi provide many of the most important elements of exercise for disabled people. For example, one physiotherapist has suggested that an ideal exercise programme for people with rheumatic conditions would include stretching, relaxation, correct body posture and what are known as 'isometric' exercises, all of which are provided by yoga and tai chi. There is also some evidence that yoga and tai chi might stimulate bone growth and strengthen bone tissue.

It is widely recognized that exercise is important for health and this might be especially true for people who are disabled. Many workers have pointed out that disability is often exacerbated by inactivity: people who have rheumatoid arthritis, for example, often avoid physical activity because of stiffness and pain; however, muscles become weak if they are not used and this can not only lead to further disability but to a worsening of joint problems. In fact, studies have shown that people with rheumatoid arthritis who exercise require less sick leave and experience less disease progression than those who remain inactive.

Another benefit of yoga and tai chi as exercises is that they allow people to become more aware of their bodies and how they move. Thus, mobility is not only improved by greater strength and suppleness, but by greater efficiency and awareness; tai chi in particular develops ease and grace in movement. Given the importance of exercise for people with disabilities, and the suitability of yoga and tai chi, it is not surprising that many disabled people who have tried these disciplines have enjoyed substantial benefits.

I noted that I could get out of the bathtub easier.

I had complete relief from pain in my left leg.

I left my splints off rather cautiously in case the pain would recur, but that was not so. Everyone I know has commented on how well I look and how much better I am walking etc.

I can type for the first time in ten years.

Breath exercises – pranayama in yoga, chi kung in tai chi – can also be particularly valuable. Yogis believe that all forms of ill-health are manifested in the breath; tai chi masters claim that effective movement is that which is in harmony with the breath. One severely disabled woman who made remarkable progress by the practice of yoga used breathing exercises as her starting point:

Having just spent several months in a coronary ward ... my breathing was so shallow as to be barely noticeable, so I played particular note of the emphasis that [was] placed on the importance of breathing correctly. This was something that I could work at even though I was so poorly.

It is also worth pointing out that most of the section on meditation (see page 147) is applicable to yoga and tai chi; see in particular the subsection entitled 'Meditation and disability'.

However, it would be a mistake to see the benefits of yoga and tai chi purely in terms of exercise for the physical body. As has already been pointed out, yoga and tai chi involve meditational and spiritual aspects which many people find to be valuable. Some find that learning a form or a set of asanas gives them a sense of achievement; others experience more profound shifts in themselves and their sense of the body.

This morning is a 'good to be alive' one. I am happier than I have ever been, and I can now enjoy a measure of good health which God, by His Grace, now enables me to enjoy . . . . It is far better to manage something than to lie in bed and get frustrated. Normally, I have been upset, which is bad for multiple sclerosis victims.

Just sitting here I feel great, very well in myself.

The section entitled 'General well-being' in Chapter 2 contains further observations on the use of yoga and tai chi by people with disabilities.

Yoga and tai chi in practice

Yoga and tai chi are normally taught to groups of eight or more, though some teachers do offer individual tuition. There are a number of different ways of locating an appropriate yoga or tai chi class. Listed below are the addresses of a number of organizations which can refer you to teachers in your area. Many adult education centres offer courses; private schools and teachers advertise for pupils in local newspapers and magazines. Access may present some difficulties in the private sector.

It has been recommended that people with disabilities should attempt to locate an experienced teacher: it is possible that certain yoga postures and/or tai chi movements might be dangerous or cause complications for disabled people if used inappropriately and modifications to the standard routine are sometimes required. You will also have to exercise care and judgement for yourself: avoid overdoing it or pushing yourself to the limit. After all, avoiding such things are an integral part of what yoga and tai chi are all about.

There are some specialized classes for disabled people; appropriate contacts are listed below. If you undertake a class with a non-specialist teacher, it might be a good idea to have some preliminary contact to discuss any special needs you might have.

Which should I choose?

It is not possible, of course, to prescribe yoga and tai chi on the basis of particular disabilities: personal preference is always key. However, some workers have pointed out that a higher proportion of yoga than tai chi exercises are appropriate for people with the most severe disabilities. Some other things you might like to think about to help you make your personal choice are as follows:

- Meditation and relaxation techniques are a more prominent feature of yoga than of tai chi.
- Tai chi might be seen as more difficult to learn: if you make a mistake or forget part of the form in tai chi, this is much more off-putting than doing so during asanas.
- Tai chi is about movement: many people prefer the idea of learning flowing, relaxed and pleasurable movements to the more static exercises found in yoga.
- The stretches and movements in tai chi are more gentle than those found in yoga.
- If you are interested in Taoist philosophy, tai chi, as an expression of that philosophy, would seem an appropriate option.
- There are more yoga than tai chi classes specifically catering for the needs of people with disabilities: moreover, yoga is perhaps easier to adapt and modify than tai chi.
- Tai chi requires more space than yoga.

It is also worth pointing out that there are various styles and forms of tai chi and yoga. There are, for example, Hatha, Iyengar and Zazen yoga and Yang, Lam and Wu tai chi. Don't worry too much about the different styles at first: it is much more important to find an appropriate teacher.

Resources

Send SAEs to the following.

Yoga

The Yoga for Health Foundation
Ickwell Bury, Biggleswade, Bedfordshire SG18 9EF.
  Tel 0767 627271.

Residential yoga courses. Many disabled people visit Ickwell Bury and there are special courses for people who have multiple sclerosis. The Foundation also publishes a list of teachers throughout the country. Some workers say that the approach of Yoga for Health involves a little too much attention to achievement and to 'pushing yourself to do it'.

You and Me Yoga Centre
The Cottage, Burton in Kendall, Cornford, Lancs LA6 1ND.
  Yoga and special needs.

The British Wheel of Yoga
1 Hamilton Place, Boston Road, Sleaford, Lincs NG34 7ES.
  Tel 0529 306851.

Iyengar Yoga Institute
223a Randolph Avenue, London W9 1NL. Tel 071-624 3080.
  Some people say that Iyengar is a more physical approach,
  with greater emphasis placed on the postures than the
  meditations.

Yoga Biomedical Trust
PO Box 140, Cambridge CB1 1PU.
  Can provide contact addresses for yoga therapists throughout the country for a £3 charge. Yoga therapists use exercises which are designed to aid the treatment of specific
  conditions.

Tai chi

Village Hall Tai Chi
163 Palatine Road, Manchester M20 8GH.
  A centre of information and advice about tai chi for people
  who have special needs.

British Tai Chi Chuan Association
7 Upper Wimpole Street, London W1. Tel 071-935 8444.

Tai Chi Union for Great Britain
Ray Wilkie, Secretary, 23 Oakwood Avenue, Mitcham, Surrey
  CR4 3DQ.

Tai Chi North
Chris Thomas, Secretary, 131 Tunstall Road, Knypersley,
  Stoke-on-Trent ST8 7AA.
  Tai chi instructors in the North of England and Scotland.

11

Orally taken remedies

Introduction to homoeopathy

Homoeopaths treat illness by using extremely small doses of common substances in pill form. In this respect, homoeopathy is much more like visiting the doctor than most other complementary therapies: the practitioner takes a case history and writes a prescription. However, homoeopathic remedies work on very different principles to conventional drugs and the case history is consequently a very different affair.

Homoeopathy was founded in the late 18th century by Dr Samuel Hahnemann. Hahnemann discovered that a dose of quinine, the cure for malaria, caused the symptoms of malaria in a healthy person and, by a series of experiments in which dilutions of various materials were used as remedies, he formulated the principle of 'like cures like'. He also noticed that, generally speaking, the more a remedy was diluted, the more effective it became. Modern homoeopathy is still very much governed by Hahnemann's basic principles. Homoeopaths believe that human beings have an inherent ability to heal themselves and that homoeopathic remedies stimulate this process. As such, they emphasize treating the patient as opposed to the disease, and they prescribe remedies depending on the particular characteristics of each individual. It is common for two people with precisely the same medical condition to be prescribed different homoeopathic remedies.

Homoeopathic medicine is generally free from unwanted side-effects and, though some say that it is hard to see why it should work, there is much scientific evidence in its favour (see 'Does it work?' in Chapter 1). It is this combination of safety and efficacy which makes homoeopathy an attractive form of medicine.

Visiting a homoeopath

The first visit to a homoeopath is generally the longest, with the initial case history taking between an hour and an hour and a half. Many people believe that just talking in depth about symptoms can be therapeutic in itself and some have commented that it is a relief to be able to say exactly what they want to about their condition. For example, many orthodox physicians might not be interested in whether an aching joint was worse in certain weathers because that information would not affect their diagnosis.

For a homoeopath, the exact details of an individual's symptoms are of prime importance and these will be asked about in detail. Other questions might concern an individual's sleeping patterns, emotional reactions or even taste in food. All in all, the homoeopath will try to make an assessment of the client's entire mental, physical and emotional state. This 'constitutional type' is the basis for choosing the most appropriate remedy.

After writing the prescription, the homoeopath will give you advice on taking the medication; for example, it is necessary to avoid coffee and camphor, and arrange for a second appointment. A course of homoeopathic treatment involves several appointments, particularly in chronic or serious conditions. The homoeopath will assess your progress at each appointment and, if needed, prescribe new remedies or 'potencies'. Different potencies reflect different dilutions of the remedy. The higher the potency, the more the remedy has been diluted and the greater the effect homoeopaths believe it to have.

It may take several tries for the homoeopath to find the right remedy; on the other hand, you might be lucky straight away and in this case, a further visit to the homoeopath might bring no change in treatment. Some people feel slightly cheated if this happens as they may have had to pay good money just to be nodded at and told to wait and see. However, that is just a fact of homoeopathic treatment.

One thing to watch out for is an 'aggravation reaction' when symptoms worsen for a few days. This is a sign that the homoeopathic medicine is working and is generally harmless. However, in certain conditions, for example, asthma, aggravations can potentially cause some difficulties and this is something to discuss with your homoeopath.

Modern homoeopaths prescribe in various ways. In 'classical homoeopathy', the aim of treatment is to find the one single remedy most appropriate for the individual, but some homoeopaths vary this by prescribing more than one remedy or by practising 'polypharmacy', where several homoeopathic medicines are combined in a single pill. One non-classical practice which can be very useful for disabled people is the prescribing of remedies to be used 'as required' for recurring symptoms. This is something worth discussing with your homoeopath. Obviously he or she will try to help you improve to the point where symptoms no longer do recur, but complete cures may not be possible. In this case, your homoeopath could prescribe remedies for you to keep and use whenever you feel a certain symptom returning. Being able to resort to a harmless and non-addictive treatment for recurring symptoms is something many people find a particularly attractive feature of homoeopathy.

Homoeopathic treatment: people with physical disabilities

For disabled people, one of the problems about homoeopathy is the theory that symptoms are good, that they express a 'fundamental disharmony in the body' and reflect the body's 'natural healing systems coming into play'. Homoeopathically speaking, it is wrong to suppress symptoms with drugs because this does not cure the underlying problem; in fact, it may add to it. Which is all very well, if it were not for the fact that for many disabled people, there may be little that can be done about the 'underlying problem' and it is the symptoms which are the distressing thing.

Nevertheless, homoeopathy can be a useful therapy for disabled people as it appears particularly well suited to a variety of common health problems of disability. The box gives details of conditions which routinely treated by homoeopaths: those marked with an asterisk* have been the subject of scientific studies in which homoeopathy was shown to be a successful treatment.

Conditions regularly treated by homoeopaths

> Muscular pains*; oedema* (swelling); irritable bowel*/constipation; urinary tract infection/cystitis*; respiratory infections*/'flu*; vertigo*; drug dependency/side-effects; poor circulation; sleep difficulties.
>
> Homoeopaths disagree on whether the following conditions are amenable to treatment:
>
> Spasticity; hypotonia (flaccid muscles); muscle stiffness other than that due to arthritis; epilepsy; ataxia (inco-ordination).

Many disabled people have enjoyed the benefits of being able to control such symptoms without recourse to potentially harmful drugs.

Homoeopathic treatment of disabling disease

People with disabling diseases can benefit from homoeopathy in similar ways to other physically disabled people (and of course, to the able-bodied too.) Improvements in general well-being and the control of problems such as constipation are commonly reported. But individuals with conditions such as rheumatoid arthritis or multiple sclerosis are also interested in the possibility that the disease process itself may be controlled by homoeopathic treatment.

Homoeopathy and rheumatic conditions

Most homoeopaths are confident of their ability to treat rheumatic conditions, and there have been a number of scientific studies which have shown that such confidence may well be justified (see also 'Does it work?' in Chapter 1, especially for some of the problems of research in complementary medicine).

One of the first trials investigated rheumatoid arthritis, comparing homoeopathic treatment with high dose aspirin. The result was positive for homoeopathy: a 65% improvement rate compared to only 14.6% for the aspirin. Two-thirds of those who improved on homoeopathy were taking no other medication after one year.

This study was fiercely criticized at the time and the authors conceded that there were a number of flaws in their trial. To support their findings, they conducted a second research project. This time, patients on orthodox 'first line' drugs were either given homoeopathy or an inert placebo. Those patients who took both conventional and homoeopathic medication improved significantly over a three month period whereas those who took only a placebo in addition to their standard drugs experienced no change.

However, some people have argued that the improvements found in the trials were fairly modest. Homoeopaths counter that trials impose rigorous constraints on the doctors involved and they claim that if they had the freedom to prescribe other homoeopathic remedies over longer periods of time, the improvements would have been more impressive.

Another successful trial involved the treatment of fibrositis and this study was particularly interesting in that the results for homoeopathy were at least as great as for any other treatment so far reported. However, one trial of homoeopathy for osteoarthritis was unsuccessful, and though some homoeopaths have criticized this study, there does seem to be a feeling that the effects of homoeopathy for osteoarthritis may not be so dramatic as for rheumatoid arthritis and other 'systemic' rheumatic conditions.

Dr Peter Fisher, who is a homoeopath and rheumatologist at the Royal London Homoeopathic Hospital, says that the effects of homoeopathy in rheumatic conditions depend on the disease duration; that is, how long someone has had the disease before coming to the homoeopath. In the early stages, it is possible to make dramatic improvements but, if the disease had progressed, there may be physical damage to the joints which will not be reversed by homoeopathic treatment. Even in these cases, however, Dr Fisher claims that homoeopathy remains a useful palliative, improving pain and stiffness and acting on the 'flu-like symptoms of rheumatoid arthritis. There is also the possibility that homoeopathic treatment may prevent, or slow down, further progression of the disease, though it can be difficult to know whether this has happened.

A fairly typical example of long established arthritis is John, who is 85 and has had arthritic problems for many years. After a course of homoeopathy he told his practitioner:

> I feel so much better in myself: my constipation is completely gone and my appetite is much improved . . . I have more energy. I am not sure what to tell you about the arthritis. My hands are a lot better but my legs are still painful. My back still hurts, though not as much, and I am still pretty stiff in the morning. One good thing is that I do sleep better.

Homoeopathy and multiple sclerosis

Though there is little known about homoeopathy and MS, homoeopaths say that they may be able to reduce the severity of some symptoms of the disease. One person with personal experience of MS has written that she finds homoeopathic remedies particularly useful for problems such as 'burning soles of feet and palms of hands'; 'aching optic nerve and aching arms and legs'; 'overtired muscles' and various other aches and pains. This woman uses particular homoeopathic remedies as and when her symptoms occur, but people who go for a course of treatment often find that it helps reduce the severity of symptoms overall.

Homoeopaths claim that people with MS who try a course of homoeopathy tend to enjoy a higher quality of life. There are a number of cases where people have been able to stop tranquillizers and pain-killing drugs and have experienced less pain and fatigue, or have enjoyed a lifting of the spirits after a course of homoeopathy. Yet in many of these cases, the physical disabilities were unaffected by treatment.

> What I am doing is not so much "curing paralysis" as helping John to overcome his dependence on drugs and reduce pain and fatigue.

Because MS is such a variable disease, few homoeopaths feel that they are able to comment on how homoeopathy might affect disease progression. Some dramatic recoveries from serious disease have been reported but it is difficult to draw conclusions from case histories and such spectacular successes are unlikely to be commonplace.

According to Dr Fisher, physicians at the Royal London Homoeopathic Hospital feel that they can reduce the frequency of exacerbations of MS. Some evidence to support this claim comes from a trial conducted in Greece in which 33 people with MS were given homoeopathic treatment over the course of two years. Whereas there had been an average of about 5 exacerbations per person in the two-year period preceding homoeopathic treatment, in the two-year period following its completion, an average of only 2 relapses occurred, a reduction of 57%. Steroid use also fell, by 62%, and psychological testing found significant improvements on a number of variables such as tension, emotional stability and self-assuredness.

There are a number of reasons why it is hard to draw conclusions from this trial. For a start, it did not conform to many of the basic standards of modern medical research: there was no control group to assess how the disease would have progressed without treatment and because both patients and physicians knew who was receiving homoeopathy, the improvements seen may have been due to the placebo effect or even biased assessment on the part of the doctors involved. Moreover, it is not clear how the patients were selected for the trial or whether there were changes in other factors (for example, diet or medication) which might have affected the result.

One interesting thing about the study was that the people who took part had had MS for an average of only six years. This perhaps gives some weight to a view expressed by a number of homoeopaths, which is that the effect of homoeopathy on the course of MS is greatest in the early stages.

Homoeopathy and other disabling diseases

There is some anecdotal evidence that homoeopathy may help reduce the severity of symptoms in conditions such as

Parkinson's disease and Paget's disease and in hereditary disorders such as Friedreich's ataxia. Little is known of how homoeopathy might affect the course of such diseases.

Homoeopathy in practice

Homoeopaths practising in the UK can be placed in one of four categories.

1. Doctors with orthodox qualifications who wish to apply for recognition by the Faculty of Homoeopathy must have three years experience as a registered medical practitioner and must pass a suitable examination. They add the letters 'MFHom' to their name.

2. A number of GPs occasionally dabble in homoeopathy, prescribing homoeopathic remedies instead of drugs in simple cases. Because they have no formal training, their ability to use homoeopathy successfully is limited.

3. 'Lay' homoeopaths are those who practise without formal medical qualifications. They generally study, part-time, for three or four years and become registered by the Society of Homoeopaths on examination by a registration committee.

4. Unregistered/unqualified 'homoeopaths'. There are, of course, people calling themselves 'homoeopaths' who are neither registered nor medically qualified. Though it is consequently hard to know what training they have, and though seeking a registered practitioner is always advised, unregistered homoeopaths are probably less dangerous than say, unregistered acupuncturists or osteopaths. Surprisingly, there are reports of a number of successes at their hands.

It is clear that anyone seriously interested in homoeopathy should either consult a lay homoeopath registered by the Society of Homoeopathy or a doctor who has the letters 'MFHom'. So, which should you choose?

Doctor homoeopaths obviously have a greater grasp of basic medicine and there are certain times when this is particularly relevant. People willing to cut down their drug intake are advised to do so in consultation with a doctor, particularly if they take steroids. Another instance when medical supervision is required is when any worsening of the condition might be dangerous. Homoeopathy often causes an aggravation of symptoms in the early stages of treatment and in a condition such as asthma or epilepsy, such an aggravation might be medically serious. Finally, if you are not sure about your symptoms, a medically qualified homoeopath can be of enormous help, especially as he or she may have access to laboratory tests, X-rays and the like. If you get abdominal pain, for example, you might assume that this was a side-effect of the drugs you were taking, or some kind of bowel problem caused, perhaps, by the stress of your new job. But abdominal pain can be a symptom of a variety of other medical conditions and a doctor homoeopath is in a good position to spot whether a particular symptom needs further investigation.

On the other hand, some people prefer lay homoeopaths. One of the main reasons people give is that they feel they can relate very naturally to a lay homoeopath whereas they find homoeopathic GPs to be much like any other doctors in terms of their relationship with their clients. For example, one woman with a spinal injury visited a medical homoeopath. Though she had gone for the treatment of a mild skin condition, her doctor insisted on discussing spasm and offered her anti-spasmodic drugs, which she had to refuse to take. Moreover, medically qualified homoeopaths often use terms such as 'spastics' or 'rheumatoid patients' whereas lay homoeopaths are much more likely to talk of particular people who have particular problems. Perhaps this reflects the view that doctors, whether homoeopaths or not, treat patients not people.

Ultimately, of course, it is up to the individual to decide whether a homoeopath's medical and scientific knowledge is more important than his or her ability to relate to clients on a natural, one-to-one basis. It is also worth pointing out that many homoeopaths, probably the majority, combine both.

Homoeopathy on the NHS

Though the majority of GP homoeopaths practise privately, homoeopathy is available on the NHS at a number of special-ized hospitals and outpatient clinics; simply ask your GP for a referral. Waiting times vary from about two months to just over a year.

Apart from cost, one of the advantages of the homoeopathic hospitals is that they offer a variety of therapies. At the Royal London Homoeopathic Hospital, acupuncture, manipulative medicine (osteopathy/chiropractic), nutritional therapy and relaxation training complement the homoeopathic work. Physiotherapy and occupational therapy are also available. In theory someone with, say, rheumatoid arthritis could go for a homoeopathic treatment, find out whether dietary changes might be worthwhile, have manipulation to improve mobility and learn some physiotherapy exercises to maintain any improvements.

The down side is that this might not be quite how it works in practice and that homoeopathic physicians working in a hospital setting might be too pressured for time to give proper homoeopathic consultations. It can also be hard to build up a relationship with a hospital doctor. Finally, of course, you might live too far from a homoeopathic hospital to make regular visits feasible.

Resources

For the location of your nearest medically qualified homoeopath, send an SAE to:

The British Homoeopathic Association
27a Devonshire Street, London W1. Tel 071-935 2163.

To find a registered lay homoeopath, send an SAE to:

The Secretary, **The Society of Homoeopaths**
2 Artizan Road, Northampton NN1 4HU. Tel 0604 21400.

For a referral to a homoeopathic hospital or clinic, simply ask your GP. Hospitals are located in Bristol, Glasgow, London and Tunbridge Wells with outpatient clinics at Glasgow, Liverpool, Manchester and Northwich (Mid-Cheshire).

HERBAL MEDICINE

Introduction to herbal medicine

Herbs have been used for healing for many thousands of years; in fact many modern drugs are based on original herbal remedies. Perhaps the best-known of these is aspirin, which contains a substance found in the bark of willow trees. Herbalists believe that by producing medicines directly from plants, they can provide a remedy which is safer, gentler and more effective than an equivalent synthetic drug.

There are a number of different systems of herbal medicine. Most cultures have developed their own characteristic form of herbalism and, in some, elaborate systems of diagnosis and treatment have evolved. Typically, herbs are ascribed certain qualities, for example, cool, bitter or stimulating, and used according to the deficiencies or excesses of those qualities in the patient: disease states believed to result from heat are treated with 'cooling' herbs; those from languor with 'stimulating' herbs and so on.

Chinese herbal medicine is a particularly interesting example of traditional herbalism. Practitioners of Chinese medicine believe that our health is determined by the flow of a vital force or energy called *chi*. This *chi* must flow in the correct strength and quality through the body for health to be maintained. Just as an acupuncturist will use needles to correct energy imbalances, so a herbalist will prescribe herbs. A number of traditional Chinese remedies have been shown to be effective by scientific trial: in one recent study, a herbal preparation was found to have a strong effect on eczema.

Modern medical herbalism tends to place less emphasis on the 'traditional' qualities of herbs. Herbalists are taught the medical actions and uses of different herbs in terms of their chemical constituents and they prescribe accordingly. However, this is not a simple case of 'one disease, one herb'. Medical herbalists take complex information about various systems of the body and build up a picture which will be different for each client they see, even for those with similar medical conditions.

Herbalists claim that the medicine they practise is much safer than drug therapy. They point out that whereas drugs based on herbal cures contain only one 'active ingredient', herbs contain many substances and so any potential toxic effect is buffered. For example, whereas the use of aspirin can lead to stomach problems, the use of willow bark rarely leads to such complications. In fact, herbalists sometimes use willow bark to treat stomach symptoms.

Many orthodox doctors have reservations about the way in which herbal medicine is practised. Some point out that boiling up a herb in water is unlikely to give a precise dose. Others say that the amount of active substance in a herb may be too small to affect serious disease: for example, replacing cinchona bark by pure quinine has had a dramatic effect on malaria in some parts of the world. That said, most doctors are willing to accept that herbal remedies can have beneficial effects on health. If herbalists' claims about the safety of their medicine are taken seriously, and there appears little grounds for scepticism on this issue, herbal medicine might well be seen as an attractive healthcare option.

Visiting a practitioner

The first visit to a herbal practitioner is generally the longest. The herbalist will take an extensive case history by asking a variety of questions regarding symptoms, diet, lifestyle and the functioning of the various systems of the body – even those which might appear to be unrelated to the problems at hand. Traditional herbalists may also use techniques such as pulse diagnosis. The aim is to gain an overall picture so that the 'root cause' of ill-health can be established.

To give an example, it is known that certain herbs contain substances which have anti-inflammatory effects. However, these herbs are not prescribed indiscriminately to everyone with arthritis. A herbalist is much more likely to take an indirect approach, perhaps noticing and treating problems of elimination such as constipation or insufficient sweating. Practitioners say that joint symptoms often improve if such treatment is successful.

Herbs can be used in a variety of different forms. In health stores, you will often find capsules containing dried herb. However, few herbalists use such preparations: most use ready made syrups (where the herb has been boiled in water, with sugar added as a preservative) or tinctures (where alcohol has been used), but it is not uncommon for practitioners to make up preparations themselves, sometimes even picking the herbs fresh from the garden. Herbs can also be used in ointments and poultices.

Herbal preparations sometimes smell unpleasant, but not unbearably so and there is often an invigorating or 'tonic' effect after taking a dose. Herbs are generally slow to act so

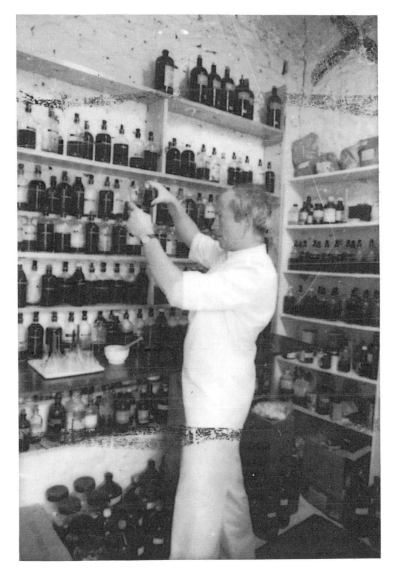

Figure 11.1 A practitioner of herbal medicine making up a remedy from a ready made herbal preparation.

practitioners are usually in no hurry to change treatment if results are initially unimpressive. However, if you are worried about the pace of progress, do discuss this with your herbalist.

Herbal medicine and disability

One of the benefits of herbal medicine most commonly reported by people with disabilities appears to be an improvement in the systems of digestion and elimination. Many herbalists are confident of their ability to control symptoms such as urinary tract infection, poor digestion, constipation or irritable bowel syndrome and this confidence appears to be justified by the experience of clients.

Indeed, the effects of herbal medicine on eczema – something which has taken on a high profile since the publication of two successful scientific trials – is explained by some herbalists in terms of elimination (the skin being one of the means by which substances are eliminated from the body).

It would be a mistake, however, to restrict herbs to the role of 'digestive tonics'. Modern medicines based on herbal remedies have actions as diverse as increasing urine production, preventing malaria and treating heart disease, and herbalists do aim to treat the full range of symptoms. For example, one herbalist has said that she is able to treat neuritis in people with MS, though she does accept that control of digestion and elimination problems also play an important role in these cases.

Some disabled people have used herbs as a direct alternative to palliative drugs:

> A cup of herb tea before retiring has replaced Mogodon [a powerful drug] to give me a good night's rest and has improved my circulation to such an extent that I have a strong pulse in my feet where none existed before.

Another set of symptoms that many herbalists claim to be able to treat are those of the rheumatic conditions.

Herbal medicine and rheumatic conditions

The fact that some herbs have anti-inflammatory or anti-rheumatic properties has been scientifically established: herbal preparations have been shown to control experimentally induced arthritis in rats and double-blind studies on humans have also demonstrated significant effects. It is also worth remembering that aspirin, one of the most frequently pre-scribed drugs for rheumatic conditions, was derived from willow bark: in fact, when aspirin first came to promin-ence, over 100 years ago, a South African doctor wrote to the *Lancet* telling the story of a rheumatoid patient who was relieved by willow bark prescribed by a Hottentot herbalist.

However, some practitioners are quick to point out that thinking of herbs as 'anti-inflammatories' or 'anti-rheumatics' may give a misleading picture. Simon Mills, a leading UK herbalist, has said:

> It is most likely that the state of scientific information about the action of herbs in rheumatic conditions falls somewhat short of the potential of skilful application ... What is apparent is that practising herbalists treat the condition often and generally have a reasonable track record in relieving symptoms.

Perhaps this reflects the view that medical herbalism is about treating people, rather than diseases. Perhaps it also explains why, for many people with rheumatic conditions, the most beneficial effects of herbal medicine have not been restricted to joints.

> You know, though the herbs haven't done much for my painful feet, they've made me feel so well in myself. I feel on top of the world!

Herbal medicine in practice

Medical herbalism

In the UK, practitioners of modern herbal medicine are represented by the National Institute of Medical Herbalism: registration follows a four-year course of training, a period of clinical practice and an examination. Members use the letters MNIMH; fellows use FNIMH.

Chinese herbalism

The Council for Acupuncture is an affiliation of five separate organizations. If you are primarily interested in herbalism, you can either contact the Council stating your wishes, or you can contact the appropriate member organizations direct. These are the International Register of Oriental Medicine (UK), the Register of Traditional Chinese Medicine and the Chung San Acupuncture Society.

Self-help and over-the-counter herbalism

Herbal medicine is also available over the counter at health stores. Self-help herbalism is unlikely to be as effective as a professional consultation. In fact, many herbalists think that the health store remedies are a travesty of true herbal medicine (see Chapter 6 for further information). You might wish to regard advice on herbalism from unqualified sources ('Aunty Agatha's Olde Herbal Advice Column') with some scepticism.

Resources

National Institute of Medical Herbalism
41 Hatherly Road, Winchester, Hants.

Council for Acupuncture
179 Gloucester Place, London NW1 6DX.

International Register of Oriental Medicine (UK)
4 The Manor House, Colley Lane, Reigate, Surrey RH2 9JW.

Register of Traditional Chinese Medicine
19 Trinity Road, London N2 8JJ.

Chung San Acupuncture Society
15 Porchester Gardens, London W2 4DB.

There is a Chinese medicine division of the British Register of Complementary Practitioners, so you can also locate competent Chinese herbalists through the Institute for Complementary Medicine (see page 276).

NUTRITION

There is probably no single topic in medicine that causes as much disagreement as nutrition. On the one hand, there are all sorts of crank diets and food fads, generally proposed as the cure to all humanity's ills. On the other, conventional physicians with minimal training in nutrition dismiss any suggestion that food might have a role in any illness except deficiency disease. Writing about food and diet brings the danger of merely adding to the cacophony of dissent. However, it does seem worth discussing some of the issues of most interest to people with disabilities.

Basic nutrition: what is uncontroversial

Human beings require nutrients such as fats, proteins, minerals and vitamins. If a person obtains an insufficient quantity of a nutrient, a specific deficiency disease may result. Perhaps the best-known deficiency condition is scurvy, which results from a lack of vitamin C and causes problems such as internal bleeding and the swelling and infection of the gums. The treatment for deficiency diseases is the provision of the missing nutrient(s) either by diet or in capsule form.

It is often stated that deficiency disease is rare in the West. Unfortunately, one of the few groups in which it might still be prevalent is people with disabilities. This is because difficulties with shopping and cooking may lead to a reliance (.. convenience foods, poverty may restrict the consumption of fresh fruit and vegetables and low appetite may limit the amount of food eaten. Finally, drugs can interfere with the use of nutrients in the body leading to an increased requirement. This has led some authorities to suggest that people who are elderly or disabled should consider supplementing their diet with vitamin and mineral pills.

In the past 20 or 30 years, it has been acknowledged that disease can be associated with excess of certain foods as well as deficiencies. Indeed, a number of studies found diet to be related to many of the major diseases in the West, including heart disease, stroke, cancer and diabetes. In the late 1970s and early 1980s, a number of Western governments set up committees to investigate the links between diet and disease and to make recommendations on healthy eating.

The results were fairly consistent: the typical diet eaten in the West is unhealthy and should be changed. The consumption of fat, especially unsaturated fat, should be reduced; the consumption of sugar, salt and alcohol should likewise be cut; fibre consumption should rise. This means that people in the West should eat more fruit and vegetables; eat more bread, cereals and potatoes; replace fatty meats with fish, poultry and lean meat; eat fewer dairy products and eat less processed food.

One of the results of such a change in diet would be a reduction in weight. Being overweight can cause special problems for some disabled people: it may interfere with mobility and, especially for those with arthritic conditions, place undesirable extra strain on joints.

Fats and oils

Everyone knows they should 'cut down on fat'. However, it is important to distinguish between two different forms of fat, saturated and unsaturated. Saturated fat is usually hard at room temperature: butter, cheddar cheese and fatty meat contain large amounts of saturated fat. Unsaturated fats are usually soft or liquid at room temperature: sunflower seed oil, fish oil and soya margarine are good examples.

Though saturated fats provide plenty of energy, they are not an essential part of the diet. Some polyunsaturated fats, however, cannot be synthesized by the body and must be taken in the form of food. These substances play a vital role in human metabolism. Some authorities suggest that there are benefits to be had from increasing the dietary intake of these 'essential fatty acids'. Modifying the diet by increasing consumption of foods such as linseeds, liver and fish and reducing the intake of saturated fats is one way of achieving this end; another option is to take a supplement of evening primrose oil (EPO) and/or fish oil (EPA).

Changing the proportion of saturated and unsaturated fats in the diet is thought to lower the risk of heart disease. Moreover, the use of EPO/EPA supplements has been found to be of benefit in a variety of conditions including irritable bowel syndrome, multiple sclerosis and rheumatoid arthritis.

Fats and multiple sclerosis

The loss of sensation and mobility in multiple sclerosis (MS) is caused by damage to the myelin sheath which surround the nerve cells and which aids the conduction of nerve signals. The myelin consists largely of fats, so it is not surprising that the fat content of the diet can affect the course of MS.

A British charity called Action for Research into Multiple Sclerosis (ARMS) has sponsored research into dietary fat and MS. They have developed a diet which is high in essential fatty acids and low in the saturated fats which block their action. In addition, it provides plenty of fibre, vitamins and minerals in the form of cereals and fresh fruit and vegetables. ARMS has found that people with MS who stick closely to the diet do better that those who complied less exactly with its recommendations: they have fewer and shorter relapses and their disability score, as measured by a special scale, increases less rapidly.

ARMS believes that, as their diet provides adequate amounts of all the necessary nutrients, the taking of additional pills or supplements should not normally be necessary. However, there is room for disagreement on this issue. It might be pointed out that not everyone is going to follow the diet precisely all of the time; alternatively, essential fatty acid supplements might be seen as a sort of insurance policy, guaranteeing optimum levels of these nutrients. A more technical argument supposes that some people with MS might have some difficulties in converting the essential acids found in foodstuffs into the form in which they are used by the body. Supplements provide nutrients in a form which is simpler for the body to metabolize and might therefore be seen as a useful addition to the diet.

In conclusion, it might be best to say that whereas the use of the ARMS Essential Fatty Acid Diet is strongly advised, the use of extra pills and supplements should be a matter of personal choice for discussion between client and practitioners. One suggestion might be for each individual to experiment with the use of evening primrose and fish oil and determine whether the results obtained are worth the costs involved. In any event, supplements should be used in addition to rather than instead of the ARMS diet. For a further discussion of the use of nutritional supplements, particularly where self-prescribed, see the appropriate section in Chapter 13 (page 217).

Fats and rheumatoid arthritis

There is strong evidence from scientific trials that diets high in polyunsaturated fat and low in saturated fat are of moderate benefit to individuals with rheumatoid arthritis. A typical diet used in such experiments involved cutting down on saturated fats by excluding cheese, milk, fatty meats etc. and increasing the intake of polyunsaturated by a combination of appropriate foods and fish oil supplements. Typical results were that trial participants did better on clinical scores such as morning stiffness and tender joint count while complying with the diet but relapsed (i.e. got worse) after returning to normal patterns of eating. Other trials have demonstrated positive benefits to EPO and EPA supplementation irrespective of dietary change.

The explanation for this effect appears to be that high levels of saturated fat aggravate rheumatoid arthritis rather than low levels, or polyunsaturated, being curative. It is not really known whether manipulation of fatty acids might have some role in the control of other rheumatic conditions.

Stimulants in the diet

Many people in the West consume large quantities of tea, coffee, cola and cigarettes as a habitual part of daily life. Each contains substances which act as stimulants on the nervous system and there is evidence which links these substances to a variety of conditions including cancer, pain and heart disease.

Moreover, as with any drug, dependence and tolerance may develop. This means that some people cannot start or get through the day without their 'fix' and they may suffer withdrawal symptoms if they go without. In general, it is worth speculating on how a person's psychological well-being is affected by the habitual use of chemicals which act on the nervous system. The increased use of decaffeinated coffee and herbal tea attests to the fact that many people feel better in themselves and much more alert once they have ceased to use large doses of stimulants as part of their daily life.

Food sensitivity

Surprising as it may sound, certain everyday foods can cause illness in susceptible individuals. This is called food sensitivity, a term which encompasses two very separate (though often confused) concepts: food allergy and food intolerance.

Some people are allergic to particular foods in the same way that others are allergic to pollen, cat's hair or cleaning fluid. When they come into contact with a culprit food, they get a reaction, such as a skin rash, almost immediately. Food allergy, like other allergies, involves the immune system.

Food intolerance is unlike allergy. The reaction to an offending food is much slower and the symptoms caused are less predictable. Whereas an allergy can be triggered by miniscule amounts of a substance (for example, by kissing someone who has just eaten the offending food), normal sized portions are required for a food intolerance reaction. Moreover, while the foods and other substances implicated in allergy are many and various, intolerance most often occurs with commonly eaten foods: wheat and milk products in the UK; wheat, milk and corn in the USA; rice and soya beans in Taiwan. The immune system is not a major factor in food intolerance; in fact, its mechanism is not really known.

Now whereas individuals with food allergy are generally aware of their condition, most people with a food intolerance do not suspect that their health problems are food related. The only way that this can be discovered is by trying what is known as an elimination diet. This has two stages: an *exclusion* phase, in which foods are avoided by using a special diet, and a *reintroduction* phase, in which individual foods are eaten once more. If symptoms are relieved in the exclusion phase, there may be a food intolerance. By reintroducing foods in a systematic way, and observing whether they cause a re-appearance of symptoms, it is possible to determine which foods are the culprits. Though it is more common for some foods to cause intolerance than others, the particular foods causing intolerance will vary from person to person. Every person found to be food intolerant has to design a personal diet which avoids culprit foods. Sticking to this diet will lead to the relief of food induced symptoms.

Food intolerance can cause many and various health problems. One of the most common conditions has been nicknamed 'Thick Note Syndrome'. An individual may complain of so many various and diffuse symptoms – bloating, nausea, fatigue, mouth ulcers, indigestion and headache – that their medical notes become extremely thick. Other symptoms associated with food intolerance include migraine, asthma, intestinal ulcers and a variety of mental and emotional disturbances such as anxiety, depression, mental exhaustion and insomnia. Food intolerance has also been linked to certain cases of epilepsy and to hyperactivity in children. In all these conditions, the method of diagnosis and cure is exactly the same: the elimination diet. Elimination diets have also been used for disabling diseases.

Food intolerance and rheumatoid arthritis

There is excellent evidence from well-conditioned trials that, for some individuals at least, food intolerance can cause or maintain rheumatoid arthritis and that elimination dieting can be an effective treatment. For example, in a study published in the *Lancet* in 1986, dietary manipulation led to a number of significant improvements. Findings included the number of trial participants in severe pain at night falling from 40% to zero, the average duration of morning stiffness falling from one hour to 10 minutes and the average degree of pain experienced in 24 hours falling by more than 60%. Moreover, there were improvements on laboratory measures such as erythrocyte sedimentation rate – interestingly enough, this is one of the tests by which rheumatoid arthritis is diagnosed. Amongst 'good responders', there were improvements on 20 out of the 22 different variables that were measured.

A number of other studies have produced similar results. Further evidence comes from successful studies of fasting, which is one possible form of the exclusion phase of the elimination diet. There have also been some well-controlled case studies and laboratory investigations.

Not everyone with rheumatoid arthritis will benefit from an exclusion diet. One of the problems of the scientific studies is that they use averages, a statistical technique which obscures the fact that whereas some individuals do very well, others experience little improvement. Estimates vary widely as to the proportion of people with rheumatoid arthritis who respond to the food intolerance approach. A survey of authorities on the subject gives this consensus: in 5–10% of cases of rheumatoid arthritis, food exclusion can have a total or near curative effect; in a further 25%, dietary manipulation leads to such great improvement that drugs are no longer required; perhaps up to half of the remaining 70% or so can be helped to at least some degree. This means that somewhere between one-half and two-thirds of people with rheumatoid arthritis might benefit from an exclusion diet.

Food intolerance and other rheumatic conditions

There have been no scientific trials of the elimination diet for rheumatic conditions other than rheumatoid arthritis. There is some anecdotal evidence that the food intolerance approach can be of benefit in systemic rheumatic conditions such as fibrositis and lupus. Generalized joint pain which has not been given a specific diagnosis is also well indicated, especially when associated with other symptoms of food intolerance (see above).

Food intolerance and multiple sclerosis

Many authorities on food intolerance do not appear to believe that food intolerance can cause the damage to the nervous system ('demyelination') which is characteristic of MS. Moreover, ARMS takes the position that the symptoms of MS are too vague and random to test by an exclusion/reintroduction diet. However, some people with MS claim to have benefited from eliminating certain foods from their diet and these claims have been popularized by lay authors such as Judy Graham and Roger MacDougall.

There appear to be three possible theories about the role of food intolerance in MS.

1.*Food intolerance cannot cause demyelination* However, a person with MS might coincidentally be intolerant to certain foods and suffer classic food intolerance symptoms such as headache, lethargy, depression and bowel problems. Many of these symptoms are similar to the symptoms of MS and this may lead to the false belief that a successful exclusion diet has lead to the relief of MS rather than an unassociated food intolerance.

2.*As (1) above except that people with MS are more likely to have food intolerance* This hypothesis is supported by a study which linked MS and sinusitis, a condition believed to be especially common amongst those with food sensitivities.

3.*Food intolerance can cause demyelination in certain individuals* At least one leading nutritionist believes this to be the case.

Perhaps it is not important which one of these theories you believe; perhaps it would even be scientifically impossible to find out which was correct. It must be up to each individual to decide whether they would like to try an elimination diet. Given that the potential gains can be large – relief from some of the symptoms of MS – and the disadvantages perhaps relatively minor – the fuss and bother of dietary change – the argument for an experimental exclusion diet in MS might be seen as a strong one.

Vitamin and mineral supplements

There are probably as many viewpoints on the use of vitamin and mineral supplements as there are people interested in health. However, there are two major ideas which seem worth rescuing from the din and clamour.

Firstly, many people are eating diets which do not appear to provide sufficient quantities of essential vitamins and minerals. A number of studies have shown that, for example, in 1980 only one in seven of the British population was eating a diet that contained even the minimum recommended allowances, and that 75% of people with rheumatoid arthritis showed evidence of malnutrition. It is also worth pointing out that other groups, for example, elderly or disabled people, might have an even lower nutritional intake or that certain groups, such as pregnant women or people who are ill, have increased nutritional requirements.

The taking of some general multi-vitamin and mineral supplement might therefore be seen as a good idea, especially for those individuals who might have a lowered intake of food or an increased nutritional requirement. This might well include some disabled people.

Another important idea is that some individuals might eat a perfectly healthy, balanced diet yet remain deficient in one or more essential nutrients. The reason for this could be because they had an exceptionally high requirement, whether due to hereditary predisposition or illness. However, such deficiencies are more commonly ascribed to defects in the body's ability to absorb and/or use certain vitamins and minerals.

Medical practitioners who subscribe to this theory test clients for vitamin and mineral deficiencies and prescribe supplements as appropriate. In certain cases, where deficiency is attributed to a serious defect in absorption, such supplements will be given by injection. Some practitioners use their successes to demonstrate that their client's illness was actually a form of deficiency disease; other practitioners make the more modest claim that once such deficiencies are remedied the body is far better able to heal itself.

Special diets

There are numerous commercially available diets each of which prescribes a set pattern of eating as a cure for all human ills. The Hay diet proposes that protein should be eaten separately from carbohydrate; the Dong diet is based on that of Chinese peasants; the Stone Age diet urges us to return to the eating habits of pre-agricultural man; the raw foods diet blames the saucepan for our modern ills. Each of these diets has a number of vociferous proponents.

> I was once on a radio program with Nathan Pritkin. We were debating the merits of which diet was better – his or mine. It wasn't really a debate but a shouting match . . . He said don't eat nuts – I said nuts are a good source of protein. He said only eat the whites of the eggs – I said only

eat the yolks etc. etc. He died of leukaemia. I contracted cancer. Two schmucks arguing over how many angels can sit on the head of a pin.

It is not surprising that these diets work for at least some people. Most are low in fat and sugar, recommend a high intake of fresh fruit and vegetables and forbid processed foods, tea, coffee, alcohol and smoking. This is all fairly sound advice and it could have important benefits for health, particularly for those with poor diets or those addicted to coffee or alcohol. Moreover, many of the diets involve complete avoidance of certain foods, often wheat and milk. People who are intolerant to just those particular foods excluded by the special diet will do very well indeed.

The problem is that the success of a diet is seen by its proponents as a vindication of the philosophy behind the diet (e.g. that the agricultural revolution was a bad idea, that proteins and carbohydrates fight). 'My diet works', the argument goes, 'and I have letters from grateful patients to prove it. This demonstrates that certain foods do in fact fight [or whatever] and that everyone should avoid eating protein and carbohydrates together'. But the individual successes of special diets might more plausibly be attributed to their exclusion of certain foods and the fact that most involve, in general, a fairly healthy way of eating.

There is no best diet for all people – only diets which suit particular people at particular times of their life. It may not be necessary to restrict your diet to some fixed pattern which is complex and which may interfere with your home and social life if there are other, simpler ways of improving your diet. On the other hand, you might find something particularly attractive about a diet.

> I went to a talk by Michio Kushi, the macrobiotic teacher. I connected with everything he said, it all made perfect sense to me, not just the diet but the whole way of life. I've eaten macrobiotic, and felt great, ever since, some 14 years. It's sometimes hard to remember that back then I was ill with what was believed to be multiple sclerosis: I haven't had a symptom for more than a decade.

See also the section on Nutrition in Chapter 13.

Nutrition in practice

One of the main problems in getting good professional advice about nutrition is that many of those best placed to give such advice, doctors and consultants, seem hopelessly prejudiced against the idea that food can be an important element in healthcare. This is a problem you might have to face with your own GP who may, for example, be unaware of the scientific evidence on food intolerance.

Moreover, the stance of major charities such as the Arthritis and Rheumatism Council is typically that 'there is little scientific evidence to suggest that allergies to particular foods can cause arthritis, except in a very few cases' and that 'low fat diets ... together with an increased intake of some cold water fish or vegetable oils ... are not likely to bring much benefit to most arthritis sufferers'. Given the available scientific data on the subject, this position can only be seen as scandalous.

There are some doctors who are interested in nutritional approaches to healthcare. The British Society for Nutritional Medicine and the British Society for Allergy and Environmental Medicine have some 500 members between them, all of whom are orthodox medical practitioners. These two organizations are a good first bet, though many of the doctors practise privately and, presumably, expensively.

An alternative might be to see a dietitian, to whom you can be referred by your doctor. The problem with dietitians is that they work strictly under doctors' orders. It is no good going to a dietitian and saying that you would like to try an exclusion diet, or nutritional supplementation, because a dietitian will only carry out a doctor's prescriptions. Dietitians can, however, be a useful resource if you want to lose weight, or if you want to make sure your diet is adequate.

Complementary practitioners and diet

Many practitioners incorporate dietary advice into their treatment. Dietary change and the use of nutritional supplementation constitute a major part of the work and training of naturopaths; herbs, hydrotherapy and osteopathic techniques may also be used. Other practitioners likely to have interest and understanding of nutrition include homeopaths and herbalists.

However, practitioners of therapies ranging from yoga to massage to healing may also sometimes give dietary advice. This might be seen as problematic; after all, practitioners of touch and movement disciplines may not have received any formal training in nutrition. Often the advice will be quite general, 'try to eat more fibre, what about a general multivitamin etc.' but if you receive more specific advice, for example, to eat a particular diet, or cut out specific foods, it may be worth asking about the reasons for the suggestion made.

Some practitioners work mainly, or exclusively, with dietary manipulation. Such practitioners may describe themselves as 'nutrition consultants', others as purveyors of 'natural health services', yet others use the label 'allergists' or 'clincial ecologists': the sheer range of different services and belief systems on offer can get quite confusing. Again, you will have to rely on your own resources to find a reputable practitioner. In addition to the advice in Chapter 4 on how to check unregistered practitioners, there are a number of things to look out for, and a number of things to avoid.

Be wary of nutritionists who prescribe a set pattern of eating as a cure for all ills (unless of course it is a diet you are particularly interested in). It is also worth being just a little bit cautious if your practitioner uses techniques not previously mentioned in this chapter. Such techniques include: hair mineral analysis; desensitization (in which minute doses of an allergen are used to cure allergy or intolerance) and the use of special machines, pulse rate or muscle strength to diagnose food sensitivity. Each of these techniques has its proponents, but there does seem some sense in being careful once you leave the mainstream – especially as there is evidence that at least some unorthodox methods of nutritional testing are inaccurate.

Finally, discuss follow-up with your practitioner. What happens once you go on a diet? Is that it for life? How will you cope with food restrictions? It is a good sign if a practitioner is willing to make allowances for any difficulties you might have in complying with a régime; be cautious if your practitioner's response is merely to bang on about the fundamental importance of diet.

Resources

The two societies for doctors interested in nutritional medicine are:

British Society for Nutritional Medicine
Stone House, 9 Weymouth Street, London W1N 3FF.
  Tel 071-436 8532.

British Society for Allergy and Environmental Medicine
'Acorns', Runsey Road, Cadnam, Southampton S04 2NN.
  Tel 0703 812124.

To obtain a consultation with a dietician, ask your GP for a referral.

People with MS interested in the Essential Fatty Acid Diet should contact:

Action for Research into Multiple Sclerosis (ARMS)
4a Chapel Hill, Standstead, Essex CM24 8AG. Tel 0279 815553.

Professional dietary advice is available on a one-to-one basis at ARMS centres throughout the country.

Organizations of complementary practitioners of nutrition

British College of Naturopathy and Osteopathy
6 Netherhall Gardens, London NW3 5RR.
Tel 071-435 6464.

Nutrition Consultants Association
51 Robinson Meadow, Ledbury, Herts HR8 1SX.
  Tel 0531 5934

The Society for the Promotion of Nutritional Therapy
2 Hampden Lodge, Hailsham Road, Heathfield, East
  Sussex TN21 8AE. Tel 0435 867007.
  Send £1 for a list of members in your area.

The main centre for macrobiotics in the UK is:

The Community Health Foundation
188 Old Street, London EC1. Tel 071-251 0831.

12

Other therapies

COUNSELLING

Introduction to counselling

Everyone experiences emotional difficulties at some point in their life and at such times it can be valuable to talk things over with someone. There are occasions when it might be most helpful if that person was a professional counsellor. For example, it is common to discuss emotional difficulties with friends or family, but if a distressing situation involves those close to us, we might want to look for someone with an independent perspective, someone with whom it would be possible to discuss matters in private. Moreover, sometimes people suffer emotional distress that friends and family do not know how to deal with, having perhaps never experienced it themselves. Again, someone with professional experience of dealing with emotional issues and problems might be an appropriate person to turn to.

The term 'psychotherapy' is often used in addition to, or in place of the term 'counselling'. Some people use counselling to refer to the provision of short-term emotional support, whereas psychotherapy is seen as going somewhat deeper, exploring unconscious issues and long-term trends. However, the two terms are seen as synonymous for the purposes of this section.

Counselling is often thought of as being practised by 'head shrinks', typically middle Europeans with bow-ties, thick accents and a tendency to inquire about a person's sexual feelings towards their parents. Most modern counselling is poorly represented by this picture: a serious chat with a wise friend or teacher would be closer to the mark. Another important misapprehension is that you have to be 'wrong in the head' before you need counselling. Many clients of counsellors might be described as 'perfectly normal, sane people'. The fact is that perfectly normal, sane people do encounter emotional difficulties and that many have been enabled to lead fuller and more contented lives through counselling.

Choosing a counsellor

There are many different traditions of counselling. Freud developed what is called psychoanalysis and it is this which conforms most closely to popular stereotypes of counselling. More recent innovations include transactional analysis, which looks at a person's relations with other people; rational emotive therapy, which concentrates on allowing a person to relinquish irrational thoughts and fears; Gestalt therapy, the aim of which is to work through unacknowledged thoughts and feelings, sometimes by using role play; and Rogerian therapy, which allows the counselling to be directed by the client. In fact, there are many more therapies than these: quite a bewildering array.

Fortunately, many modern counsellors learn a range of methods and practices and select what is most suitable for each client on an individual basis. So it is unnecessary to take the trouble of working out which particular theoretical approach you like the sound of and trying to find a local adherent. What is more important is to find a counsellor who feels right for you, someone you feel you can trust completely, whose manner towards you seems accepting and understanding.

Most reputable counsellors will set up an initial interview so that you can get a feeling of whether they suit you. You might want to ask a little bit about your counsellor's style. Some counsellors incorporate techniques other than talking into their work, for example, dream analysis, role play and psychodrama (acting out difficult situations), body work (such as massage, movement or breathing exercises) or drawing. It is important that the methods your practitioner will be using are ones you find appropriate and suitable.

This initial meeting also gives an opportunity to discuss what you want out of counselling. You will have to consider whether your aim is short-term support, perhaps to help deal with some immediate crisis, or whether you would like to explore deeper and longer-term issues, such as your family, upbringing and background, and the overall trends and patterns in your life.

For example, Al's girlfriend leaves him just before an important set of exams. Al rings a telephone helpline to discuss his difficulties; the counsellor is supportive and suggests some things which might help Al cope with the next few weeks. Later in life, however, Al finds himself continually frustrated by his relationships. He contacts a private counsellor: the sessions start by focusing on Al's family and background with the hope of seeing how early experiences might have informed Al's relationships as an adult. Al's use of a helpline just before his exams is an example of counselling providing short-term emotional support to help coping with a specific problem; Al's visits with a private counsellor are an example of the deeper uses to which counselling can be put.

The first meeting with a counsellor also gives you a chance to discuss issues such as how often you would like your appointments, and – something which is particularly important – at what point you might feel that you could bring counselling to a close, or at least, what goals you hope to achieve in the short-term. It is worth remembering that the point of counselling is not to provide a crutch upon which you will eventually become dependent, it is to allow you to take more control over your life, to become more independent.

It might be difficult to know any of these things at the outset. How is a person to understand what he or she wants out of counselling without getting counselling first? However, the point is not so much that you need these things absolutely sorted out in your mind before you start, but that the way in which you are able to discuss these things with your counsellor will help you decide whether they are right for you. It is a good sign if you feel that your counsellor is able to deal constructively with problems such as the aim and end goal of your counselling.

Some workers have suggested that you should see at least two or three counsellors for a first interview before deciding. What is paramount is that you feel free to say yes or no to each counsellor; you are the buyer, and you must feel comfortable with them (see also 'Choosing a practitioner' in Chapter 4).

Counselling is perhaps too complex an issue to be dealt with in a book of this nature and if you want to know more, it might be worth reading a more specialist text (see the 'Further reading' section).

Counselling and disability

There is increasing acknowledgement that some of the emotional problems faced by disabled people need special recognition and attention from counsellors. For example, the British Association for Counselling has recently set up a Disability Issues Sub-Committee to develop interest in and information about counselling for disabled people. Another recent innovation is what is known as 'peer counselling' which is when counsellors for disabled people are disabled themselves. One group which supports peer counselling put it like this:

> Our own experience tells us that it does help to talk to other disabled people . . . who have faced some of the difficulties we face.

However, many people who work in the area of counselling and disability are at pains to point out that there is nothing inherent in being disabled that necessitates counselling. Dr Mike Oliver, Lecturer in Special Needs at Thames Polytechnic, became disabled as a young man:

> There's an assumption that because something happens to someone's body which requires medical intervention, something inevitably happen to one's mind as well, and this requires psychological intervention. Many disabled people are depressed [or angry] not because of some intrinsic connection with their body not working, and therefore their mind not working, but because of the social circumstances and limitations that occur as a consequence of being disabled. If you'd been living at home for two years and couldn't get into your own lavatory, you'd be angry. If you'd applied for 54 jobs without getting a single interview you'd be depressed.

Counselling can start to address some of the fear, anxiety, depression and anger that can result from having a disability. It can also address the personal and sexual problems that some disabled people face. It is also worth pointing out that a significant part of all counselling (whether involving disability or not) consists of the attempt to unravel the influences to which we have been subjected, influences which very often prejudice our ability to make decisions. Many of these influences involve other people's attitudes towards us. In fact Carl Rogers, an important figure in counselling, has written an essay consisting entirely of the comments a child might be subjected to as an everyday part of growing up: 'You're clumsy'; 'You should be a lawyer'; 'Boys don't like clever girls'; and so on. However, many of the messages that we receive are indirect; for example, though a man might verbally express his love for his wife, his behaviour might imply something very different.

One particular version of counselling, called psychosynthesis, involves exercises designed to counter these influences directly. Clients are asked to repeat statements such as 'I have a body, but I am not my body' or 'I have emotions, but I am not my emotions'.

Other counsellors work in different ways, however. One technique is to explore and challenge a client's beliefs. For example, by careful questioning, one counsellor discovered that part of one man's problem was that he thought he would never have a girlfriend again. The counsellor discussed this with the client and attempted to make him more aware of his own thinking. It became apparent that the man was having employment difficulties as a result of his arthritis and he believed that to have a girlfriend you needed 'money, a house and a fast car'. The counsellor explored this issue with the client, asking if every man he knew who had a girlfriend was rich and drove a car. The client had to accept that this was not the case and this went a little way towards resolving his fear and anxieties about sex and relationships.

Julia Segal, who has extensive experience of counselling people with multiple sclerosis, says that the condition brings with it a number of difficult emotional issues. These include grief, denial, loss of social role and status, loss of control and independence, death and difficulties with sex and relationships. She says that counselling can help people explore these problems. Often they find that what is causing the most distress is not the problem itself, but their way of thinking about the problem.

A successful series of counselling sessions might help you gain insight and understanding of your life and set out your options for change. It will give you the ability to deal with things better in the future. What counselling will not do is solve all your problems and make you feel universally wonderful. Nor will it change the world: for example, counselling has enabled some disabled people to come to terms more readily with the stigmatization and prejudice that they face; it has not made that stigmatization and prejudice go away.

Counselling in practice

Counselling can take place in a number of different contexts. Almost all complementary therapy involves some informal counselling and a number of practitioners have realised the importance of talking and have taken appropriate short courses. Many clients have found this informal counselling to be an extremely valuable, if unexpected, part of treatment.

However, if you are particularly interested in receiving counselling, you will probably be best off looking for a more specialist service. Private one-on-one counselling offers the most intimate and intense setting, one which is likely to be conducive to an explorative and challenging experience; at the other extreme, group situations offer a more social and supportive situation (see also 'Group situations' on page 62). This is especially true of self-help groups. In marriage or family counselling, a couple or family will receive counselling at the same time.

The telephone has made counselling much more accessible, and perhaps somewhat less threatening. A number of disability organizations run help lines which are staffed by trained counsellors: many are freephone, others will call you back if you are worried by the thought of a large bill.

Some counsellors and counselling services specialize, for example, in marriage problems or addictions. Though most counsellors deal with a range of problems, you might want to consider seeking specialist help if your problem is very specific.

Like many of the therapies in this book, there is no set number of sessions for counselling. Counselling needn't be a long-winded process: one telephone counsellor has been quick to point out the usefulness of the 'one-off' call, perhaps to discuss a crisis. However, it is likely that serious or long-term difficulties will require a greater investment of time, thought and energy.

Another point that many practitioners like to stress is that counselling should end at some point. Counsellors shouldn't be used as crutches, and hard as bringing things to a close can be, the point of counselling is, after all, greater self-reliance.

Resources

For private counsellors in your area, contact:

British Association for Counselling
37a Sheep Street, Rugby, Warwicks CV21 3BY. Tel 0788 578328.

Specialist services

CARE
Arlington Park House, Sutton Lane, London W4 4HD.
Tel 081-994 0578.
Counselling centre specializing in disability and long-term illness.

Derbyshire Centre for Integrated Living
Long Close, Cemetery Lane, Ripley, Derbyshire DE5 3HY.
Tel 0773 742165.
Specialist peer counselling services available.

Cerebral Palsy Helpline
Tel 0800 626216.
Telephone helpline.

Spinal Injuries Association
Tel 081-883 4296.
Telephone helpline.

Action for Research into Multiple Sclerosis (ARMS)
London – 071-222 3123.
Glasgow – 041-637 2262.

Birmingham – 021-476 4229.
24 hour telephone counselling service.

The Association to Aid the Sexual and Personal Relationships of People with a Disability
286 Camden Road, London N7 0BJ. Tel 071-607 8851.
    Provides appropriate leaflets and operates a telephone counselling service.

RELATE Marriage Guidance
Herbert Gray College, Little Church Street, Rugby CV21 3AP. Tel 0788 573241.

The Samaritans
Check your phone book for your local group's number.
    24 hour telephone helpline, but specialist counselling is not available.

HYPNOTHERAPY

Introduction to hypnotherapy

One of the themes of this book has been that public perceptions of complementary therapies often differ significantly from the reality of healthcare as practised. Perhaps there is no case where this is more true than hypnotherapy, about which there are two prevalent misconceptions.

Firstly, hypnosis is not, as it is widely believed, some kind of occult state; in fact it is possible to fall into a trance quite naturally as part of everyday life. Perhaps the best known example of this is when car drivers notice that they 'wake up' at the end of the journey having no recollection of having travelled from A to B. The mechanisms of hypnotherapy are similarly everyday. For example, telling someone that they 'look great' has a markedly different effect to asking them whether they are ill. Hypnotherapists use suggestion in the same way as you or I would as part of daily life: they just do so in a much more purposeful and coherent way.

The second misapprehension about hypnotism is that it involves falling into the power of a charismatic (and potentially evil) other. Even when induced by a therapist, all hypnosis is self-hypnosis: it is about self-control, not about control by someone else. A corollary is that hypnosis will not make a person act out of character, or do something to which they would otherwise object.

In practice, hypnotherapy is often used as a self-help technique. The point of visiting a practitioner is not so much 'being hypnotized' but learning how to hypnotize oneself. Once in a hypnotic state, suggestions can be used to achieve various goals. For example, the suggestion that 'my hand feels cool and free of pain' can be used for pain relief. Everyone has heard of the 'power of the mind': perhaps hypnotherapy might best be thought of as a tool to access that power.

Hypnotherapy can be used for both physical and psychological problems. Some practitioners use hypnosis primarily as an aid to psychotherapy. The trance state, so it is said, eases the exploration of the unconscious and allows difficult issues to be dealt with without the 'resistance' which occurs as a normal part of non-hypnotic psychotherapy. Hypnotherapy can also be used to deal with problems such as pain, insomnia or bowel symptoms. Though treatment of these conditions often involves some counselling or psychotherapy, the problem itself is not exclusively psychological. The main focus of this section is the use of hypnotherapy for physical symptoms.

Visiting a practitioner

After taking an appropriate case history, the practitioner will spend much of the first session explaining a little about hypnotherapy in general and about the treatment that will be given. This is often an opportunity for the practitioner to emphasize the self-help nature of hypnotherapy.

Often, a simple exercise will be used to demonstrate suggestion. For example, the practitioner might use suggestion so that a client raises an arm without being aware of doing so. The practitioner might also make a more formal assessment of 'hypnotizability' – in which there appears to be some sort of natural variability – and may also make use of psychological testing. Later sessions will be given over to the teaching of self-hypnotic techniques. A course of hypnotherapy is often surprisingly short: three or four sessions are often sufficient to introduce and teach hypnotic techniques.

Hypnotherapy can also be taught to groups. Hypnosis is induced by the use of a relaxation technique and appropriate suggestions made to the group as a whole. For example, a group for people with irritable bowel syndrome was asked to imagine a smoothly flowing river. In these situations, the distinction between hypnotherapy and creative visualization (see page 150) becomes increasingly blurred. As such, you might also want to read the section on 'Meditation, relaxation and creative visualization' if you are interested in hypnotherapy.

Hypnotherapy and disability

In common with meditation, hypnosis can be deeply relaxing and revivifying and it can be used for this purpose alone. However, the real power of hypnotherapy lies in the use of suggestion, the words and images employed during the trance to bring about a healing effect. As such, the potential applications of hypnosis are limited only by the imagination.

An interesting case of an imaginative use of hypnotherapy involved a man who found it difficult to wear an artificial leg because he experienced profuse sweating at the amputation site. He was taught self-hypnosis and used suggestions such as 'I feel a cooling breeze on my leg' to remedy the problem. The use of hypnotherapy for irritable bowel syndrome (mentioned above) involves a similar use of suggestion tailored to counter a specific problem and, for this particular condition, hypnotherapy has been shown to be a successful treatment by well-controlled scientific trials.

Hypnotherapy has also been widely employed in the treatment of chronic pain. It is worth remembering that hypnotic anaesthesia was practised many years before the advent of ether. Suggestions of numbness and coolness, or warmth and relaxation, can be used according to the type of pain experienced, and this can be an especially powerful technique if used daily at home.

Hypnotherapy in practice

The organization representing orthodox physicians who practise hypnotherapy is one of the best-respected in the UK and there are a number of reasons why consulting a doctor hypnotherapist might be preferable to visiting a non-medical counterpart. In the first major survey of complementary medicine, the practice of lay hypnotherapy was one of the few areas which the authors found particularly worrying: one complaint was that the distinction between psychotherapy, hypnotherapy and self-help was often insufficiently clear. Another group has pointed out that there is a particularly large number of training institutions and registering bodies and that standards vary widely. The conclusion must be that consulting a non-medically trained hypnotherapist is something which should be approached with caution and you should use the advice on checking unregistered practitioners given in Chapter 4.

Resources

For medically qualified hypnotherapists contact:

British Society of Medical and Dental Hypnosis
42 Links Road, Ashtead, Surrey KT21 2HJ. Tel 0372 273522.

For 'lay' hypnotherapists try:

National College for Hypnotherapy and Psychotherapy
12 Cross Street, Nelson, Lancs.

UK College of Hypnotherapy and Counselling
10 Alexander Street, London W2 5NT. Tel 071-727 2006.

There is a hypnotherapy division of the British Register of Complementary Practitioners, so you can also locate competent individuals through the Institute for Complementary Medicine (see page 276). Given the poor state of regulation in hypnotherapy this might be seen as a useful resource.

MISCELLANEOUS THERAPIES

The first two therapies listed in this section are worthwhile practices but fall outside the scope of the book. The remainder are included because there are reasons to suggest that they might best be avoided.

Art therapies

Art therapies divide along the traditional distinctions between different artistic forms. There is music therapy, dance therapy, drama therapy and art therapy itself, which, when used in a specific sense, refers to painting, collage and sculpture.

In work with people with learning disabilities, artistic therapies can be used as a medium of learning and social interaction. A popular theory is that the use and training of intuitive forms of expression and communication may pave the way for the learning of more complex, abstract and culture dependent systems of information exchange.

Most of the usage of artistic therapies with people who are not learning-disabled can often be described as psycho-therapeutic. Painting and drawing may aid the expression of unacknowledged beliefs and emotions; in dance therapy, it is postures and movements which give form to the unconscious. In either case, it is believed that mental and emotional problems can be dealt with more effectively and constructively once they have been given a physical form. For an example, see the use of art therapy with cancer patients on page 55.

Some practitioners, however, see art therapies in much more simple terms: creativity is healthy, and whether somebody sings, draws or dances, the act of expression will itself be health promoting.

Biofeedback

A biofeedback machine gives us information about our body that we would not otherwise be able to obtain. This information can then be used to help us regulate functions which are normally beyond our control. For example, a biofeedback device might measure a person's heart rate and display it in the form of a line on a computer screen: the longer the line, the faster the heart beat. With practice, people can learn to lower their heart rate by making a conscious effort to change the computer display and after a while they will be able to do this without having to be hooked up to the measuring instruments.

The use of biofeedback machines by physiotherapists is increasing, especially in the USA. In disability work, they have been used to regulate continence, decrease spasm, control muscular tension and even promote correct posture and walking in children with cerebral palsy.

Biofeedback tells us much about the body's ability to self-regulate: practitioners of complementary medicine sometimes point to biofeedback experiments to explain how their therapy might work. Biofeedback has not been included in the main body of this book because it is a complex technique which uses high technology and which does not involve a medical philosophy similar to that of other complementary therapies. Most of the biofeedback which is available outside conventional medical establishments focuses on changing the patterns of brain waves and thereby allegedly inducing a meditation like state. As such, it is closer to the 'New Age' than to a healing technique.

Therapies to be wary of

Radionics

Radionics is the best-known of the therapies which use 'black boxes'. Practitioners believe that 'energy patterns' are emitted by living organisms and that disharmonies and distortions can be identified and corrected using a special machine, basically a type of electronic device without electricity. Practitioner and client do not need to be physically near to each other for therapy to take place, in fact, the whole process can take place by post.

At best, radionics is distant healing using a physical object, the black box, to unlock intuition and focus healing powers. At worst, it represents the lunatic fringe of complementary medicine. It is hard to think of any advantage of radionics over other complementary therapies.

Healing objects: crystals, pyramids and magnets

Though there can be little harm in someone spending a few pounds or dollars on a crystal or a magnet from their local health store, visiting a 'crystal therapist' or a 'pyramid healer' is a different matter. Apart from the fact that the practitioners claim they are successful, it is hard to see what such therapies have to offer and it would be wise to consider other ways of spending time, effort and money.

Note, however, that some practitioners of healing use magnets or crystals as objects for their clients to focus and dwell upon. Such healers do not refer to themselves as 'magnet therapists'. See also the section on 'Acupuncture' for a description of the use of magnets on the acupuncture points.

Applied kinesiology

Also known as 'touch-for-health', this form of therapy was developed by chiropractors in the USA and posits that different illnesses affect a person's muscle strength in characteristic ways. Diagnoses are made by asking the client to push against a resistance provided by the practitioner. Because such a technique is highly prone to fudge and suggestion, applied kinesiology would seem to require exacting standards of professionalism, training and registration. These standards do not appear to have been met in the UK. Moreover, there have been two scientific studies which appear to disprove the claim that kinesiology can be a useful diagnostic technique.

Iridology

Practitioners of iridology believe that they can diagnose illness by searching for characteristic markings on the coloured part of the eye. However, there has been a scientific test of iridology which appears to disprove it: iridologists who were shown photographs of the eyes of people with gall bladder disease were unable to distinguish them from photographs of the eyes of healthy volunteers.

The New Age

The New Age is a catch all term to describe a philosophy which incorporates innovations in lifestyle, health and culture. What distinguishes New Age therapies is that, because they form just one part of a larger enterprise, it is difficult to use them independently from that enterprise. New Age therapy often entails taking on a whole new belief system and unfortunately, that belief system is, at the current time of writing, somewhat less than coherent. It includes ancient herbal formulas; subliminal 'I can make mega-money!' tapes; corn circles; non-invasive music; reincarnation; rebirthing; encounter therapy and a number of variations on fringe psychotherapy; rituals; celestial attunement; crystals and ecological politics. New Age therapies include colour therapy, pattern therapy, astrological therapy, reincarnation therapy, various types of spiritual healing and the aforementioned fringe psychotherapy. The aim of the New Age is nothing less than complete personal and social enlightenment.

Most New Age therapists fail on most of the criteria set out in Chapter 4 on how to find reputable practitioners. There is no particular reason to think that any of the New Age therapies work. If you are personally into the New Age, if its philosophy makes sense to you, then a New Age therapy might be a good choice. If you are not a believer in the New Age, and if you see medicine as a practical business, you might be best off putting time and effort into something else.

Part three

Complementary
healthcare in practice

13

Self-help

Many people feel the self-help aspect of complementary medicine to be a positive advantage: to take an active part in the healing process is seen by many to be an empowering and liberating experience. Many professionals believe that treatment starts to become most effective when clients shrug off the passive role as a 'recipient of therapy' and become actively engaged in their own healthcare.

A discussion of the relationship between professional help and self-help in complementary healthcare can be found in Chapter 1. To recap briefly: if an individual has a serious problem with his or her heatlh, treatment should involve a professional medical practitioner. Competent professionals have experience and understanding of healthcare and this puts them in a good position to give advice; they should be seen as 'enablers' who help individuals to achieve their aims, rather than 'experts' who take power over others' lives on the authority of technical knowledge. An ideal situation is when client and practitioner manage to form a 'therapeutic partnership' in which, as in any relationship, mutual trust, empathy and respect are key elements. Self-help has many advantages, and it often plays an important role in complementary therapy, but it should be seen as an additional resource.

Walk into a book shop or health store, however, and the message is very different. It is easier to sell a product (be it a book or a pill) if it claims to provide a cure than if it claims to play a small part in a long and difficult healing process and, as a result, many simple 'quick fix' cures are advertised. Complementary healthcare takes time, focuses on healing rather than cures, does not make exaggerated claims and treats individuals, not diseases (which is why a 'herbal pill for arthritis' makes little sense). Many see the self-help books

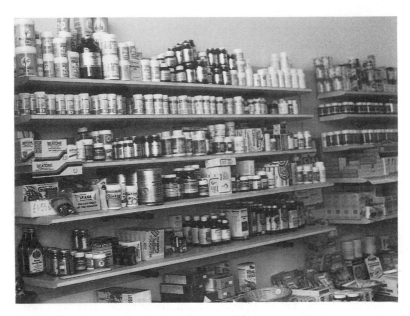

Figure 13.1 The inside of a health store. The message seems to be that healthcare can be 'do-it-yourself', and that the support and advice of an experienced practitioner is not needed.

and pills found in health stores as a travesty of true complementary practice. On the other hand, for some disabled people, difficulties of money, time, transport and access can make self-help at home seem a more attractive option than visiting a practitioner. Perhaps it is best to see self-help as a useful resource, albeit one which must be approached with some caution.

This chapter will focus on the self-help available from health stores and book shops or, perhaps, that suggested by friends. A practitioner will often suggest self-help techniques, and self-help is the important part of disciplines such as tai chi or yoga: the concern here, however, is health activities which are engaged in without the involvement of a professional. This is sometimes described as 'independent healthcare' or even 'do-it-yourself healthcare'. Listed below are sections on diet and nutrition; orally taken remedies (homeopathy, Bach flower remedies, biochemic tissue salts); herbal and folk remedies; aromatherapy; yoga, tai chi and meditation and psychotherapy. It is suggested that, where possible, you read the major sections devoted to these therapies before reading about their use as self-help. There are also a number of general points worth bearing in mind.

- It is unlikely that remedies bought off the shelf will make a major impact on any individual's state of health. Many people have found that such remedies have been useful for mild skin conditions, colds, bruises, shock and upset and the like. Cases in which an individual has overcome a major and long-term health problem in a similar way are extremely rare.
- When buying health products, it is better to do so on the advice of a friend, a professional or a book than to do so by asking a salesperson (who is unlikely to be qualified to dispense such advice) or by reading the sales blurb on the product itself (which is unlikely to be balanced).
- Beware of claims such as 'proven' or 'guaranteed results': the more a product offers, the less it is likely to deliver.
- Orally taken remedies have to be used in certain ways. For example, you must stay clear of coffee while taking homeopathic medicaments. It is best to make sure you have such information available: a good book can be invaluable here.
- If you make any major changes to your lifestyle, for example, a change of diet or a new exercise programme, inform your GP (though see 'GPs and diet' on page 229 and 'Nutrition in practice' on page 191).

Health books

Most books on complementary healthcare are written primarily because the author has some point to make. Typically, a practitioner will discuss the use of the therapy they practise and they will obviously want to show it in the most positive light possible. As a result, only the most successful cases are normally included and little mention is made of the limits, failures and problems of the technique in question. Many books are crammed with miraculous stories and letters from grateful ex-patients telling heart warming stories of overnight cures. Always bear in mind that the function of such books is to put across the author's view of things ('My therapy is absolutely wonderful') and to make the publisher a profit ('Buy this book, it'll change your life'). They do not give a good insight into the actual experience and practice of complementary health-care. Perhaps this is why so many books make healthcare seem such a simple business.

An associated point is that many books relate individual stories: someone overcomes their cancer or multiple sclerosis using say, a certain diet, concludes that this diet is then the cure for everybody's cancer or MS and so writes a book to spread the doctrine. One of the most famous examples of this is Roger MacDougall, author of *My fight against multiple sclerosis*. MacDougall is now a vigorous campaigner for a certain diet he developed to overcome his own MS and his works contain not only large numbers of miraculous case histories but also a number of reflections on disease, the medical profession, diet, treatment and modern civilization. Remember illness happens to individuals: in complementary healthcare, it is not possible to extrapolate from 'my personal experience of MS' to 'how MS should be treated'.

Reading books about health is undoubtedly worthwhile (and the numerous suggestions for further reading in this book would be a good place to start) but it is worth bearing in mind that most books paint an over-simplified and over-positive picture of complementary healthcare. One exception is self-help books on controlling chronic pain: these are generally fair, realistic and helpful.

Finally, remember the advice given above and in Chapter 1 about the limits of self-help and the need to involve a trained professional in overcoming serious health difficulties.

DIET AND NUTRITION

There are three major reasons why changes in diet are considered by disabled people: firstly, to lose weight, something which is often recommended to people with physical disabilities as lower weight decreases the risk of a number of diseases and may aid mobility: secondly, for the relief of minor symptoms such as headaches or eczema and for greater general

well-being; thirdly, to overcome disabling diseases such as
multiple sclerosis or rheumatoid arthritis. Before reading on,
it would be worth checking the section on 'Nutrition' in chapter
11.

There are several reasons why individuals wishing to make
dietary changes are advised to do so in consultation with a
practitioner rather than by following a text. Appropriate
professionals have an understanding of the minimum basic
requirements and how they can be met, the complex way in
which foods and drugs interact and the relationship between
different types of foodstuffs. A professional can also offer
advice on how to comply with a diet most easily and most
accurately. In addition, a professional practitioner will understand that some disabled people have quite specific dietary
needs. For example, some wheelchair users require a low
energy intake coupled with a high allowance of essential
nutrients. See the Resources listings in the 'Nutrition' section
of Chapter 11 for information on how to find appropriate
professional advice.

The reasons not to see a practitioner are the traditional ones
of time, expense, transport and access. Some people are also
worried by the lack of a single co-ordinating body for nutrition professionals and by the confusing array of different
'schools' of nutritionists each with a particular story to sell.
If you do decide to change your diet by following the advice
of a book or a friend, here are some things to bear in mind.

Diets to lose weight There exist vast numbers of different diets
which are claimed to lead to weight loss. Some are published
as best selling books, others are printed in magazines. Many
regimes involve the taking of special products like milkshakes,
teas, or special biscuits, some involve the use of diet suppressant drugs. A large number of these diets are aimed at people
who lose weight for reasons of personal appearance rather than
for medical reasons and, perhaps as a result, many involve
a degree of moralizing: food is seen as temptation, eating as
failure, weight loss as virtue. Few, if any, of these diets account
for the needs of disabled people.

Perhaps most damning of all, many of the diets do not
work: weight lost during the diet is often regained at its end
leading to repeated, and addictive, patterns of dieting. One

American book summed up the problem with the phrase
'Dieting makes you fat'.

That said, there is little doubt that paying attention to diet
can help bring a person towards a healthier weight. Two special
things to consider if you do decide to go on a self-help diet
to lose weight are that weight loss should be slow, no more
than 1 or 2 lbs a week, and that products such as biscuits or
milkshakes, liquid diets and appetite suppressant drugs should
be avoided.

*Diets to overcome minor symptoms and improve general well-
being* Most people are now aware of the link between diet and
health and this had led many to try changing the foods they
eat. Theoretically, experimenting with different diets, and
seeing which personally suit you, is a good idea. In practice, however, what often happens is that certain foods, for
example, chocolate, cheese and cakes, are labelled as 'bad for
you' and avoided, whereas other foods, for example, bran,
raw vegetables and rice, are labelled 'good for you' and cooked
up with no thought given to dietary balance. Again, a strange
morality can get twisted up with food: chocolate, cheese and
cake can become objects of temptation to be resisted by the
strong or eaten guiltily by the weak ('I know I shouldn't');
conversely, eating well becomes a sign of virtue and purity
('I was such a good girl: I only ate a baked potato and salad
for lunch').

This has been encouraged by a number of commercially
available diets which, typically, prescribe a set way of eating as the answer to all mankind's ills. The Hay diet suggests
that carbohydrate and protein are eaten separately; raw
food diets prescribe large amounts of raw vegetables with
certain types eaten together ('Never eat brassicas with root
vegetables'); dairy-free and gluten-free diets suggest cutting
out either milk or wheat products. Having read the book,
people often feel that they 'ought' to follow the diet, especially as the authors will be quick to point out the perils
of non-compliance compared to the healthy, happy and
contented life which will follow from eating as they suggest.
This is often the cause of agonies of indecision over whether
that beloved tuna sandwich, or beans and rice, is really worth
it.

Many authorities will tell you that there is no 'best diet' for all humans, only diets which suit individuals at particular times of their life. Some people find they achieve great well-being by following the Hay diet or any number of others featured by diet books; others are not so lucky. If you wish to experiment with your diet, and to see what suits you and what doesn't suit you, then all well and good, but it might be seen as advisable to avoid moralizing your food, to practice 'moderation in all things' and to remember that there are few foods which can be viewed as universally 'bad' or 'good' outside the context of the diet in which they are eaten.

Finally, many working in the field of complementary healthcare are coming to believe that if a diet is good, it will be also one that you want to eat. Many people have found that, once their health has found some sort of balance, they tend to like the things which make them healthy and dislike those which agree with them less. If you sigh as you sit down to something you feel you ought to eat, or frown at the thought of what you are missing, you probably haven't got it quite right yet. (Craving certain foods is an exception to this; some people crave foods which cause them troublesome symptoms.)

Diets to overcome disabling disease There is a discussion of the relationship between diet and chronic illness in the 'Nutrition' section of Chapter 11. In the Resources listings there is information on how to get balanced professional advice on such diets. If you have a disabling disease and wish to try changing your diet, but do not wish to consult a professional, try one of the diet books listed in 'Further reading'.

Nutritional supplements

It is probable that many disabled people do not receive adequate amounts of essential nutrients such as vitamins, minerals and essential fatty acids. This is because difficulties with shopping and cooking may lead to a reliance on convenience foods, poverty may restrict the consumption of fresh fruit and vegetables and low appetite may limit the amount of food actually eaten. Finally, drugs can interfere with the use of nutrients in the body leading to an increased requirement. This is why, for many disabled people, the taking of a nutritional general supplement providing vitamins and minerals might seem a wise precaution. Moreover, there is some good evidence that essential fatty acid supplements such as fish oil and evening primrose oil can be of benefit in certain conditions (see the section on Nutrition in Chapter 11).

It is probably unwise to self-prescribe supplements other than essential fatty acids or a general multivitamin. This is because nutrients work in complex combinations, and taking a supplement of one nutrient may actually lead to a deficiency in another. It is important to take supplements regularly at the stated dosage: they should not be 'popped' informally. Most important of all, if you are taking drugs, it is essential that you consult your GP before taking nutritional supplements because drugs and nutrients can interact in potentially dangerous ways. Caution is also advised if you are on a special diet as these are often designed to provide large amounts of certain nutrients: additional supplementation could conceivably lead to an overdose, though it is not known whether this has happened in practice.

ORALLY TAKEN REMEDIES: HOMOEOPATHY, BACH
FLOWER REMEDIES, BIOCHEMIC TISSUE SALTS

There are numerous different types of pills and liquid medicaments available at health stores. In the section on Homoeopathy, it was pointed out that homoeopaths may prescribe different remedies for individuals who have the same medical condition. For example, someone coming to a homoeopath with rheumatoid arthritis may be given any one of 20 or 30 remedies: the homoeopath will choose exactly which depending on the idiosyncrasies of the condition – such as how it is affected by the weather – and of the client – such as his or her taste in food.

This makes it difficult for an untrained person to choose an appropriate remedy, and though there are books and leaflets to help, these give only vague approximations of a proper homoeopathic case history. Moreover, whereas a homoeopath will prescribe pills in a variety of different 'potencies', only one potency is generally available at health stores.

This is why, for serious problems, choosing a homoeopathic remedy 'off-the-shelf' is really no substitute for a consultation with a trained homoeopath. However, many people have found self-help homoeopathy to be useful for minor symptoms which, though distressing, may not be considered worth a visit to a practitioner. For example, one elderly man who had had polio has found homoeopathic *Arnica* very useful for muscle pain and bruising from falls; a woman with MS has written that she uses a variety of different remedies for symptoms such as burning sensations, aching muscles and pain in the optic nerve. That said, some homoeopaths will prescribe remedies to be taken as required for recurrent minor symptoms (see page 167) so it might be argued that the role of self-help in homoeopathy is limited.

Unlike homoeopathy, the Bach flower remedies is not a system of medicine which requires trained professionals. Dr Bach, the originator of the method specifically intended that the remedies be prescribed and used by lay persons. Dr Bach believed that certain states of mind, for example, apprehension, apathy or irritability, could not only hinder recovery, but might, in themselves, cause sickness. His remedies, which are prepared from the flowers of wild plants, are used to treat these underlying moods rather than the physical complaints which stem from them.

A large number of people, including a surprising number of orthodox medical practitioners, swear by the Bach flower remedies. One of the remedies is known as 'Rescue Remedy' and has a particularly large number of enthusiastic proponents: people who have taken Rescue Remedy say that it has a calming effect, decreasing anxiety and inducing calm.

The Bach flower remedies are well suited to self-help: they are simple, harmless and inexpensive and can be used as an addition to any course of therapy.

Biochemic tissue salts are another remedy found on the shelves of health stores. Although these are homoeopathic preparations, their use is dictated by an entirely different set of principles: disease is seen to stem from inadequate cell nutrition, cures are achieved by supplying the appropriate tissue salts.

During World War I, there were about fifty doctors in the UK using biochemic tissue salts: it is doubtful whether there are any today. Evidence for the salts is said to come from case histories, but these appear unconvincing to a trained eye.

Suffice it to say that money spent on biochemic tissue salts might seem to be money better spent in other ways.

FOLK AND HERBAL REMEDIES

There are many books which advocate traditional and herbal remedies for various complaints and most of these remedies are either easily made up at home or readily available over-the-counter in health stores. Many professional herbalists, however, are unhappy with the idea that individual herbs are advocated as cures for specific diseases: true medical herbalism involves the taking of a complex case history, the matching of remedies to individuals and the use of herbs in carefully judged mixtures. Moroever, scientific studies of the effects of some of the most popular off-the-shelf remedies have not demonstrated any significant effect.

Despite the unproven and irregular nature of commercially available folk and herbal remedies, most are simple, cheap and harmless (for example, two tablespoons of honey and cider vinegar in a glass of water with meals for arthritis). Still, herbs should be treated with care: some do contain toxic substances and there have been reports of poisonings following the ingestion of home-made herbal preparations.

One folk remedy which has gained some acceptance is fruit juice for recurrent urinary tract infection: cranberry juice and vitamin C tablets are believed to prevent these infections by affecting the acidity of the urine; orange juice reverses this effect and should be avoided. There is also some evidence to suggest that peppermint oil can be useful for irritable bowel syndrome. On the whole, it seems that self-help herbal medicine is better suited to 'secondary' problems, particularly those of the digestive and urinary tract, rather than to the direct treatment of disease.

If the idea of herbal cures attracts you, finding out about and using herbal remedies has little to condemn it apart from perhaps cost. It might also be worth taking the simplistic claims of some of the herbal health books with just a bit more than a pinch of salt: if you do decide to try feverfew tea, or a liver flush mixture, do it for yourself, not for someone trying to sell a magazine or book. Finally, beware of over-using any herb.

AROMATHERAPY

Aromatherapy oils can be used in various ways in the home. They can be burnt in a special burner to release their smell, they can be used in baths, they can be added to poultices and they can, of course, be made up into massage oils. As well as creating lovely smells, many people also feel that using essential oils in their day-to-day lives makes 'health' and 'healthiness' a part of their environment. As one elderly woman who had osteoarthritis put it:

> It's almost as if the oils act as a reminder that there are healthy things in life too, that life isn't just pills and injections and doctors and pain and feeling bad. I make a point of having a bath with a few drops of essential oil in it whenever I can. It is something I can do for myself and it makes me feel wonderful.

However, it is important to remember that essential oils are powerful and potentially harmful substances, so it is necessary to approach their use with a little caution.

Some general guidelines are: buy good quality essential oils either mail order or from reputable health stores; avoid anything associated with 'health and beauty' products. Some caution is advised in the use of essential oils: they should never be used 'neat' without the use of a carrier such as air, water or massage oil. Never use more than ten drops of essential oil in a burner, five in a bath, one or two in a poultice or ten drops in 30 ml of massage oil. Certain oils – rosemary, fennel (sweet), hyssop, sage, wormwood – have been associated with epilepsy and should be avoided with individuals at risk. These and other contraindications (for example, oils which should be avoided in pregnancy or skin conditions) can be found in any good book on aromatherapy.

RELAXATION, MEDITATION, YOGA AND TAI CHI

People who want to learn disciplines such as meditation, yoga or tai chi normally do so by attending a weekly class with a professional teacher and practising daily at home. Though this is the ideal way of learning such techniques, there are many simple and effective relaxation techniques which you can teach yourself.

It is generally agreed that, though you can learn meditation or relaxation without going to a class, it would be effectively impossible to learn tai chi without working in person with an experienced practitioner. Yoga is somewhere in between: it is possible to learn something about yoga from a book, a friend or a tape, but a working knowledge really requires classes from a trained teacher. See 'Further reading' for books on relaxation, yoga and meditation.

DO-IT-YOURSELF PSYCHOTHERAPY

There are three types of do-it-yourself psychotherapy. Firstly, there are a number of general books which discuss, for example, some of the typical origins of relationship problems and some of the ways in which such problems can be addressed. Such books are very popular and many people have found them to be both interesting and useful. But no matter how valuable these books can be, they cannot really substitute for direct contact with a counsellor or psychotherapist. If you have some serious worry or problem, a book may not be enough to help you.

The second type of do-it-yourself psychotherapy book consists of questionnaires, games and puzzles, the purpose of which is to give you an insight into your 'real' nature. For example, you might answer a set of questions such as: 'Do you often cross the road and leave friends standing on the other side?' or 'Do you run up the stairs rather than waiting for the lift?' and depending on your answers, the book will assess you as either a 'go-getter' or 'laid-back'. Such tests can be fun to do, but it surely does not take an expert to realize that they are of little therapeutic value.

In addition, few of the major popular texts on psychotherapy issues mention disability in significant detail: the two questions quoted above might give you some idea of the difficulties that a disabled person might find from reading a standard book of do-it-yourself psychotherapy.

The third type of book on do-it-yourself psychotherapy is worthy of particular attention. Recently, there has been an upsurge of interest in the role of the mind and the emotions in disease. A number of books have been published on this subject, some of which are excellent. However, the link between the mind and disease is an issue which must be approached with some delicacy. Not only does this mean that you should be wary of the many books which fail to do so, it also entails that even the very best books must be read with some care.

The role of the mind and the emotions in disease is discussed in various sections of this book. See in particular the section on complementary medicine and disabling disease in Chapter 2 (page 26) and the sections on family involvement and obstacles to healing in Chaper 7 (pages 239 and 243). Put briefly, there is evidence which links an individual's state of mind to the state of his or her health. In the case of serious or life-threatening diseases, those individuals who hold a more positive image of themselves, of their treatment and of life in general, and who take personal responsibility for their health care tend to do better than those who resign themselves passively to their fate. Studies such as the one which found that elderly people are much more likely to die just after a birthday than at other times of the year further demonstrate that human beings have a great capacity to keep themselves alive and healthy.

The problem comes in interpreting these ideas. In Chapter 2 it was pointed out that feeling positive, and coming to take active responsibility for healthcare, often happens quite naturally as part of the process of complementary health-care. Many of the books, however, take a much more blunt approach. For example, Judy Graham's self-help guide on multiple sclerosis contains the advice that people with MS should fight off negative attitudes and try to build up their self-esteem: 'It is important to try and keep hold of a positive body image'. In one of Elizabeth Kubler-Ross's books, there are two lists of responses to loss: 'healthy' and 'natural' responses – such as sadness – and 'unhealthy' and 'unnatural' responses – such as depression or resentment. The gist of this part of the book is that you should try and have the former type of emotion rather than the latter.

Unfortunately, it is probably no more possible to decide to change your emotions than to pick yourself up by your bootstraps. To use an analogy: you can't instantly decide to be happy because you read somewhere that happiness is a good thing. What often appears to happen when people read such books is that they just end up feeling guilty: 'Not only have I got a problem, but I've got the wrong attitude to my problem. What kind of awful person am I?'

Another set of problems is connected with the fact that psychological theories of illness can appear to 'blame the victim'. Some people have become very distressed at the thought that they may have caused themselves to become ill or prevented themselves from getting better. To make matters worse, many of those who link the mind to disease emphasize personal responsibility for healthcare. Though this is generally to be applauded, it does make it possible to think: 'If I am responsible for my health and if I am ill, that means that I am at fault.'

Moreover, if someone's health deteriorates, it becomes possible for them to take this as a sign of moral failure. This feeling can be exacerbated by reading about those 'health super-achievers' who do well. Bernie Siegel's books are packed with stories such as that of the 78 year old gardener who survived having turned down chemotherapy for his cancer on the grounds that it was spring and he ought to be making the world a beautiful place. Or the woman with motor neurone disease who came to love her wasting body, forgive her parents, control her emotions and embrace sexuality as a sacred and ecstatic form of self-expression. It is not hard to see how such stories can lead to the feeling 'I'm getting worse: I'm not good enough'.

Another belief that you may find in some books (and perhaps expressed by some practitioners) is that disease is associated with certain personality types. For example, Louise Hay describes the probable cause of multiple sclerosis as 'mental hardness, hard-heartedness, iron will and inflexibility'; other authors have discussed 'the asthmatic personality'. There are a number of reasons why the concept of 'personality traits' for certain chronic illnesses might do more harm than good.

Firstly, it is generally true that if you look for a certain personality characteristic in a person, you will often find it. For example, in the 1950s, the theory that parents determine their children's behaviour came to prominence. This theory predicts that parents of autistic children should behave in similar ways and sure enough, workers began to discuss 'the mechanicalness of human contact' of these 'refrigerator parents', a trait which was seen to cause the emotional disorder in their children. Needless to say, most people now recognize that parents of autistic children form a good cross-section of personality and behaviour. Another good example is that normal, healthy volunteers who checked themselves into psychiatric institutions as part of an experiment were described by staff as having a number of obsessional behaviours. The second reason to be suspicious of the idea of 'disease personalities' is that many of the personality traits alleged to be associated with disease are very common. For example, 'hides emotional neediness behind a facade of self-reliance' might describe most people in the UK. Thirdly, it is always possible that personality traits are an effect rather than a cause of a particular condition.

In general, the theory that certain personality types are associated with disease probably goes further to 'blame the victim' than any other in medicine. It suggests that because you are who you are, you will get disease. It also appears to have little therapeutic value.

To sum up, though many people have found great inspiration from those books which discuss the links between mind and disease, it is possible to find some of the ideas quite distressing. If anything you read about this subject does worry you, remember that it is difficult to draw simple conclusions about individual cases from general theories and that, in this context, guilty feelings are rarely either appropriate or helpful. It must be remembered that bad things do happen to good people, that you can do all the right things and still have deteriorating health. The link between the mind and disease is something which should be used as a resource to get better, not as a vehicle to lay blame.

Summary

If you have a serious health problem, treatment should involve a professional practitioner. Independent health care has some advantages but it has to be approached with caution. Certainly, the miraculous successes you read about in books are unlikely to reflect general experience: self-help might make you feel good, or help you overcome minor ailments, it will not, of itself, overcome major health difficulties. When deciding on a self-help approach, choose something that strikes a chord with you rather than something which someone else says ought to make you better. If you make any changes to your diet or lifestyle, liaise with your GP.

14

What happens in complementary healthcare

Earlier sections of this book have been concerned with the information you need before actually starting a course of complementary treatment. Chapter 3 attempted to answer the question 'What should I expect from complementary healthcare?' Chapter 4 looked at how to make decisions about complementary healthcare and Chapters 5–12 gave you the information needed to make those decisions. This chapter is concerned with complementary healthcare once it has begun, once you have actually contacted a practitioner and are about to go for a treatment session.

YOU, YOUR DOCTOR AND YOUR COMPLEMENTARY PRACTITIONER

How best to liaise

Many people seem to picture complementary and orthodox practitioners as engaged in some kind of war, at each other's throats and putting each other down at the slightest opportunity. The reality is pretty much the opposite: complementary practitioners are aware of the powerful resources of modern medicine and not only are most GPs receptive to the ideas of complementary healthcare, but a majority actually refer patients to appropriate practitioners. So if you are considering complementary healthcare, you should not be frightened of raising the subject with your GP. Moreover, there are a number of reasons why it is wise to do so.

The most general point is that your GP holds some responsibility for your healthcare and so it is important to keep
him or her aware of your health plans. After all, if you visited
a consultant at the hospital or went for a test, your GP would
keep a record of this. It is much easier to keep up a good
relationship with your GP if you are open and honest about
your health, and what you intend to do about it, than if
you sneak off to the homoeopath hoping to keep it all a
secret.

There is also the possibility that some future medical
decisions might depend on your doctor knowing that you have
had treatment from a complementary practitioner. For
example, if you are given a new regime of drugs, your
doctor will be keen to see how you progress in order to
decide whether a future prescription would be worthwhile.
Obviously, an accurate assessment of the effects of a treatment
must take into account any other treatments taking place.

This might also affect other people. The 'good citizen' reason
to tell your GP about complementary therapy is that by
matching what treatments people have had with how their
health changes, doctors will be better placed to make decisions
about healthcare in the future, decisions which might include
complementary medicine. If you have a good experience
with a complementary practitioner, telling your GP may result
in others enjoying the same benefits. If you have had a
bad experience, it can be important for your GP to know
this too.

One of the most important reasons to liaise with your GP
on complementary healthcare is the issue of prescribed drugs.
Reduced need for drugs is commonly reported by people who
try complementary therapies and though cutting down drug
intake can often be beneficial, it has to be done carefully.
Steroid preparations in particular need careful supervision,
since sudden withdrawal of steroids can lead to very serious
illness. Likewise, antibiotics have to be treated with care, as
leaving a course of antibiotics uncompleted can lead to resistant
infections. Even if you wish to cut down on other medications,
your GP may still be a source of help. For example, rather
than merely taking less of your current prescription, your GP
might be able to offer you a lower dosage pill or a switch to
a milder drug.

Finally, many people are glad to be able to check with their GP that the treatment suggested by a complementary practitioner is sensible, particularly changes to diet and lifestyle.

Liaising with your GP is not difficult: simply ask your complementary practitioner to drop him or her a note. Small changes in drug intake of medications you take 'as required' or minor modifications to diet or lifestyle can also be dealt with by post. However, if you are considering large changes to diet, lifestyle or medication, or if you want to cut down on drugs you take regularly, it would seem a good idea to make an appointment.

GPs and diet

> The issue of diet is one of the biggest stumbling blocks to effective liaison between complementary and conventional practitioners. It appears that many GPs have poor training in nutrition and it has not been unusual for GPs to warn patients off a sensible dietary change. For example, though the importance of nutrition in the treatment of multiple sclerosis is reasonably well established, few people have received suitable advice from their GP on this issue and some have even been dissuaded from making appropriate modifications to their diet.
>
> If your GP disagrees with you about a dietary change, ask whether they have any evidence that the diet would be harmful. It can be useful to point out that, in the final analysis, dietary considerations are a personal matter and that the role of the GP should be to act as a guide to prevent any overtly dangerous course of action. You might also like to mention that medical understanding about the role of nutrition in disease is constantly changing and that there are few 'established truths' in the subject.

Complementary and orthodox practitioners: what can go wrong?

Despite the fact that many orthodox and complementary practitioners enjoy a good working relationship, examples of blind prejudice do occur. For example, one man who successfully tried acupuncture was advised by his doctor to 'stick the needles back into the practitioner' next time he went for a session. On the other hand, complementary practitioners have been known to encourage people to stop exercise programmes on the grounds that 'physiotherapy is bad for you.'

Practitioners exhibit prejudice in predictable ways. In general, conventional doctors who are prejudiced believe that all complementary therapies are forms of quackery and witchcraft. They will insist, quite wrongly, that there is no evidence that any of it works and may go on to give examples of particularly ludicrous practices hoping to tar all of complementary healthcare with the same brush. Complementary practitioners who exhibit blind prejudice tend to believe that they have some sort of monopoly on compassion, seeing orthodox practitioners as heartless scientists engaged in some kind of weird, egotistical power trip. The failings of conventional medicine, such as drug side-effects, and its shortcomings, such as its neglect of the psychological aspects of health, are blown up till they encompass the whole of modern medicine, obscuring most of its positive aspects. Weird and wonderful explanations may be given as to why particular conventional treatments are bad for you.

Blind prejudice of this sort is annoying, and certainly far from constructive, but it is only a major problem if pressure is placed on you by one practitioner to ignore the advice of another – for example, if a naturopath tells you to stop your drugs or if a physician tries to dissuade you from homoeopathy. There are two things to remember when pressure of this sort is brought to bear. Firstly, it is your health that is in question and it is you who is employing the professional, so you should be as free as possible to make whatever decision you think best. Secondly, health professionals often know less than they think: if a doctor tells you authoritatively that there is no evidence that complementary therapies have any effect, he or she is speaking from ignorance (see 'Does it work?' in Chapter 1 and the Bibliography). If a complementary practitioner tells you that physiotherapy is bad for you, or tells you to stop taking drugs, he or she is being similarly uninformed. Asking the grounds on which such assertions are made ('How can you be so sure?') can often help. In either case, explain calmly and assertively why you have made a certain choice about your healthcare and emphasize that it is your health, and your decision, that counts.

Finally, avoid 'half-way houses'. If two practitioners suggest different things, don't nod passively to both and then, for example, only stick to half the diet, or only take the pills every other day. If you decide to compromise, you need to ask a practitioner's advice on how this can be done.

It is obviously better, however, to avoid having your practitioners contradict each other than to have to sort the situation out once it has arisen. It is probably no great matter to have a hospital consultant berate your choice of homoeopathy during your visit once a year, but a GP who consistently disagrees with the decisions you make, or who puts pressure on you to change them, should probably not remain your GP. (Under the current system, however, changing your GP can sometimes prove extremely difficult.) Likewise, there are lots of complementary practitioners to choose from, and anyone who makes you feel uncomfortable about your orthodox treatment is not worth your time.

One problem you will have in interpreting this advice is how to decide what constitutes 'unfair pressure'. There is often all too fine a line between opinion and persuasion, particularly where professional pride is involved. For example, it would be perfectly acceptable for a practitioner to say:

Look, you've been taking antibiotics for all this time and yet you still have your problem. I really don't think that your pills are doing much. Why not go back and talk it over with your GP?

It would not be acceptable for them to say:

Drugs are bad for you and they are not doing any good. I think you ought to come off them right now.

The areas in between are a matter of personal judgement but it is worth considering whether any advice you get is in the form of information, given so that you can make the decision, or whether it merely reinforces the advice giver's professional position and world view.

However, even with the most open, honest and unprejudiced practitioners, situations may still arise when you will be given conflicting advice. This can seem particularly difficult when it happens but it also presents an opportunity to re-affirm who is in charge and for whose benefit all this is taking place.

If you get conflicting advice (in fact, if you get any advice you are unsure about) it can be a valuable exercise to write down all the possible outcomes, both good and bad. Then write down the likelihood you give of each particular outcome occurring and just how good or bad it would be if it did. Above all, it is necessary to question the practitioners closely, asking the reasons for their advice.

Finally, real problems between orthodox and complementary practitioners are the exception rather than the rule. The overwhelming majority of cases involve, for example, someone who is taking drugs going for a massage and this leaves little scope for interference or problems. Throughout this book it has been stressed that the therapies mentioned are complementary in nature and can be used with orthodox medicine without conflict.

YOUR RELATIONSHIP WITH YOUR
COMPLEMENTARY PRACTITIONER

The relationship you have with your complementary practitioner will probably be very different to any experiences you might have had with conventional doctors. It is a common perception that doctors keep a 'professional distance' from their patients, something which normally involves a big desk, a profound lack of eye contact and a strictly formal, businesslike approach to conversation. Examinations are similarly 'professional', generally taking place with cold hands and unpleasant implements. Moreover, doctors are frequently seen to fail to ask what it is that patients really want from their visit perhaps engaging in 'symptom censorship', choosing some symptoms as important whilst ignoring others. Finally, many people say that, as patients, they are rarely allowed to choose between alternative treatments. It is not unknown for doctors to possess signs saying 'Compromise means doing it my way'.

Of course, there is a reason for all this: the relationship most conventional doctors have with their patients is well suited to the type of medicine they practice. Things are often different in complementary healthcare; after all, it is hard to retain a professional distance when you are giving someone a massage. Complementary practitioners tend to be much less formal than their conventional counterparts: first names tend to be used and conversation is more chatty than businesslike. Complementary practitioners rarely sit behind desks, if they need to take notes they tend to sit side on to the client at a table. Time is also a big factor. Due to the present imperfection of the NHS, the average GP consultation lasts between six and ten minutes and so there is often a sense of rushing to get things done or said. Most sessions with complementary practitioners last upwards of 45 minutes so proceedings tend to take place at a more relaxed tempo.

Often there will be discussion centring on what the client really wants from treatment and a number of different alternatives may be presented. Finally, complementary practitioners rarely edit their clients' accounts of their lives and symptoms. Many people find this affirmation of their experiences to be valuable.

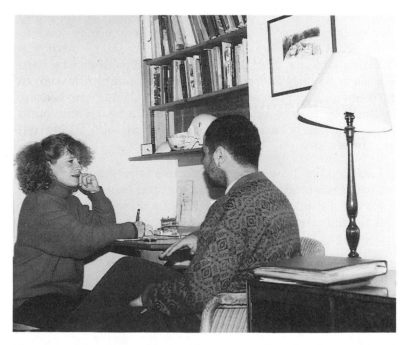

Figure 14.1 Complementary healthcare generally takes place in relaxed and informal settings.

All in all, relationships with complementary practitioners tend to be friendly and natural and many find this to be one of the most positive aspects of complementary health-care.

Your input

Of course, all relationships are two way and one thing which complementary practitioners ask of their clients is a high degree of client input and responsibility for treatment. This entails a number of things. Firstly, your practitioner may ask you a number of far reaching questions about your lifestyle, health and general temperament; sometimes this is a necessary part of diagnosis, sometimes such things come up during the talking and discussion which is a large part of many complementary therapies. The onus is on you to provide careful, accurate and honest answers and this may involve some degree of self-examination and awareness.

It is a widespread belief that complementary therapies involve the process of self-exploration. People may come to learn about themselves through complementary medicine. Learning is active, and learning about yourself can be hard work, particularly if there are things you might not want to think about. But it can also be rewarding. David, who became a wheelchair user as a result of MS, visited a healer and found that a large part of each session was taken up with talking and and discussion:

> I realized just how out of perspective I had got things, how I had concentrated on the negative, and even brought it on myself. I think I now see my life in a more balanced light. It is quite a relief.

Is there anything special I should tell my practitioner?

Many practitioners of complementary healthcare have limited experience of disability and it is important that you tell your practitioner as much about yourself and your condition as possible. In this respect, it can be a good idea to jot down a list to take along with you to your appointment as it is easy to forget things once you are there. Some things worth mentioning include:

- The basic medical facts. Some practitioners may be unaware of what exactly cerebral palsy is or what happens in multiple sclerosis. You might also want to explain symptoms such as spasm or urinary urgency.
- If you are using a therapy which involves hands-on work (for example, massage or osteopathy) it is important to spell out any difficulties you might have with spasm. Discuss any physical positions which cause spasm and mention parts of the body which are sensitive to touch.
- Certain techniques should be avoided in certain disabilities: tell your practitioner about any 'contraindications' you may have read in this book.
- A number of practitioners have had problems of 'overstimulating' when they have worked with some disabled people. It is always possible to create problems by causing changes to occur too fast but this is much more likely to happen if a system is weakened in some way: imagine stirring a cup of tea with the same force that you use to stir a pan of beans. This is not to say all disabled people are weak, it is merely to relate the observations that many disabled people have encountered difficulties because their practitioners tried to do too much, too quickly. Mention this to your practitioner and encourage him or her to go slowly and gently at first.

Something else you will be expected to do is to communicate your feelings to your practitioner. If you are worried or doubtful about anything the practitioner does or suggests, it is very important to raise this.

> I was very uncomfortable lying on the couch, but I didn't say anything because I thought this was some special position necessary for the treatment. Eventually I told him it hurt to lie down flat and he said that was no problem, we could work in a different way.

Likewise, if you want to talk about your progress, whether you think it good or bad, do so. The success of complementary healthcare depends to a great extent on good communication between client and practitioner. It is important that the practitioner knows just what you are feeling and, most vital of all, it is essential that you are not left with unresolved doubts.

Your practitioner may also ask you to make decisions about your treatment. These might be trivial ('Which arm would you like me to work on first?') but they might have important effects on your life. For example, you might be offered a number of different diets, each of which would vary in the degree of effort you would be required to make.

The most active part of complementary treatment comes with the diet and lifestyle changes you may be asked to make. You may have to cut certain things out, either as part of a diet, or because they interfere with treatment (for example, coffee negates the effects of homoeopathy). You may also be asked to practise certain exercises at home. Obviously this is a major feature of yoga, tai chi and relaxation/meditation; in fact, there is little point in visiting a practitioner of these disciplines if the hour a week is all you do. Similarly, Alexander technique involves learning new ways to use your body and it is important to apply the principles you learn with your practitioner in daily life. However, osteopaths and chiropractors may teach you some stretches and other practitioners may show you relaxation or movement exercises.

It is important that you commit yourself to complying with diets, lifestyle changes and exercise regimes. But complying does not mean a blind following of orders. It is important to negotiate with your practitioner on the changes he or she suggests you make. Discuss what you would enjoy doing most, what things you would and would not find it possible to do and any difficulties you might have.

It is all too common for things to go wrong. For example, a practitioner suggests a diet which the client will have difficulty in following. Yet instead of pointing this out, the client meekly accepts that this is the right thing to do. But after perhaps a few days of the diet, the difficulties get too much and he or she goes back to other foods. What can make matters even worse is if the client starts feeling guilty, thinking that somehow the health problem must be his or her own fault as he or she is not even able to follow a simple diet. If the client ends up feeling too guilty or stupid to admit to the practitioner about not sticking to the diet, disaster can result. Either way, little is achieved by agreeing to diet or lifestyle changes which will be difficult to make.

So be open and honest about any difficulties you think you might have in following a course of treatment. No matter how trivial you think a problem might be, remember that the practitioner is there to serve you, not to be obeyed, and that he or she may have experience of similar problems and so might be able to suggest an appropriate solution or compromise. It might also be worthwhile erring on the safe side, agreeing to a moderate set of changes you know you can cope with rather than more drastic measures you are not quite sure about.

Finally, one of the most important ways you can make an input is to turn up to your appointment in good time and to avoid making arrangements for the period immediately following treatment. Practitioners say that few things ruin a session more thoroughly than having a flustered client turn up in a hurry, or having them worry about making their next appointment when they should be relaxing and concentrating. Give yourself, say, half an hour before a session to unwind and an hour or more afterwards to let your body take stock of itself. Do not eat a heavy meal or engage in activity likely to be depleting (for example, giving blood) on the day of your session. A serious commitment to healthcare does not necessarily imply a large commitment of time and setting aside periods for you appointment and keeping these clear from other distractions is a minimum requirement of those wishing to benefit from complementary healthcare.

The 'sick role'

The first images of healthcare that many of us are presented with are those found in children's books. Typically, the scene portrayed is that of a patient lying passively in bed, with a doctor or nurse standing over them with stethoscopes, thermometers and bottles of pills. A typical caption might read: 'When you get ill, you go to the doctor and he makes you better'.

So from an early age, we are taught that we are made well by doctors and that our role is this process is passive. Moreover, we are taught that cures are total: the patient in the children's book is often shown returning to a completely normal life after a stay in hospital.

> Members of the medical profession often unconsciously adopt this picture of sickness and health and enforce it in their work. People who have received medical care for many years may be accustomed to a certain way of being treated by health professionals.

> I found that I had MS by sneaking a look in my medical records. When the consultant found out, he pulled me into the corridor and started shouting at me. He told me that my notes were none of my business.

On the other hand:

> Many of my patients just want me to write them a prescription: they shy off any discussion of lifestyle or emotional problems.

When people have a health problem, they often adopt the 'sick role' which has been subconsciously taught to all of us from an early age. This not only means being a passive recipient of healthcare ('Whatever you say, Doctor') it can also entail being a passive recipient of life ('I'll stay at home in bed because I am sick, and that's what sick people do').

Successful use of complementary healthcare involves shrugging off the 'sick role': it is important that you do not see the practitioner as a mechanic who fixes your body or see medicine as a process separate form the rest of your life. To avoid the sick role, many authorities stress that you should attempt to:

- Take responsibility for your healthcare and recognize that it is your job to take the decisions.
- Play an active role by making changes to your diet or lifestyle and by practising exercises assigned by your practitioner.
- Consider your own coping resources. If you have a serious or long-term problem, it is unlikely that any form of medicine will make you 100% better. Coping with a health problem or disability, and making the best and most positive life out of any situation, is not something that someone else can do for you; it is something which will be up to you and you alone.

Two examples of client involvement in complementary healthcare

Phyllis received reflexology at a day centre she used. The practitioner, John, asked what foot she would like worked on first. Phyllis said she didn't mind, after all, 'You're the boss'. John replied that it was her choice not his, but Phyllis again insisted, 'You're the boss'.

John arranged chairs and cushions and asked if Phyllis was comfortable. She said that it didn't matter, the most important thing was for John to have a good position to work from. On being asked why she had chosen reflexology, Phyllis said that one of the workers at the centre had suggested it: 'Everything they tell me to do I do; I don't mind anything they do to me'.

Phyllis obviously has a very passive attitude. She is unwilling to take much part in her treatment seeing the reflexology as something that was done to her. Phyllis' progress was not marked: 'I can't tell whether it helps or not'.

Compare Christine who chose to try Alexander technique. After the very first session, she started practising at home with her family and she asked her practitioner to lend her books about Alexander which she read and enjoyed.

After a few weeks, not only were her husband and mother helping her practise, they were actually joining in, with Christine teaching them what to do. She was particularly keen to emphasize that the Alexander technique was something she was learning to do so she could actively help herself, rather than having to rely on drugs.

Christine benefited enormously from her Alexander sessions, vastly decreasing her drug intake while experiencing improvements in pain, mood and energy levels. Her walking improved and she felt a return of interest in life, and her feeling of control over it.

Family involvement

The involvement of Christine's family is particularly interesting. Many practitioners have noticed that if a person's family is involved, treatment tends to be more successful. The ideal situation is where the family share similar beliefs about which practitioner and therapy would be best. Where lifestyle or diet changes are required, the family agrees on a particular course of action and works together to ensure that the changes are easy to make and that exercise programmes are maintained.

If another family member also agrees to make changes, this is best of all. Other family members don't have to do just the same as the family member who is visiting the practitioner; they could do something entirely different like taking up running or starting to go for massage. What is paramount is that other family members do things for their health and personal development.

One practitioner has reported that if a parent brings in a child for treatment, he always works on the parent first. He explains himself like this: overcoming a health problem involves change. Change is only possible when space for change is made by the people with whom an individual shares his or her life and the best way for such people to allow another to change is for them to change themselves. So the most effective way to help one family member to overcome health problems is for all family members to experience change, either by visiting a practitioner of complementary healthcare, modifying their diet or lifestyle or even just taking up a creative hobby.

Psychologists give a similar explanation in different terms: family members, they say, learn to play certain 'roles' and often someone wishing to modify their role will come under subtle pressure not to do so from the rest of the family. One of the roles people sometimes learn to play is the 'sick role', with other members perhaps taking on a 'caring role'. Because roles are difficult to change, such situations may complicate the task of achieving greater well-being. In Christine's case, the family helped to modify their caring role by taking part in Alexander exercises and, as Christine was teaching them how to do this, she too changed from her role as 'the person who needs looking after'.

You may have already heard about family roles in sickness and health. Some people find these ideas make them very uncomfortable and they worry that, somehow, they may have caused themselves or their relatives to become ill or prevented them from getting better. It is actually quite difficult to draw simple conclusions about individual cases from general ideas about psychology and, in this context, guilty feelings are rarely either appropriate or helpful. It is important to think about families and family roles as a resource to use in getting better, rather than as a place to lay blame. (See the section in Chapter 13 on 'Do-it-yourself psychotherapy' for a further discussion of this subject.)

The point should also be made that the term 'family' is taken here to refer to the people with whom you share your life. These may not necessarily be spouses, children and/or parents.

WHAT CAN GO WRONG OR CAUSE DIFFICULTIES IN COMPLEMENTARY HEALTHCARE

People rarely have significant problems with complementary healthcare, but two sorts of things can go wrong. Firstly, side-effects from treatment, though rare, are not unknown. These are given in Appendix 3. Secondly, the relationship between client and practitioner may become difficult.

Of course, minor disagreements are inevitable in almost any relationship. More often than not, these should leave you with little to worry about. One thing which can cause problems though is if your practitioner disagrees with you about what progress is being made:

He kept telling me: 'You look great! You're doing fabulous!' In fact, I looked, and felt, like a dried up prune.

It is probably okay for this to happen once or twice, after all, in the early stages of some treatments, an aggravation of symptoms is a sign that treatment is working. Moreover, changes which happen slowly can be difficult to notice on a daily basis: in some cases the practitioner is acting very much like the grandparents who tell a teenager: 'Haven't you grown!'

However, if your practitioner's assessment of your progress is consistently better than your own, this can be a danger sign. It is worth bringing this issue out into the open and challenging your practitioner's optimism, for not only do disagreements about progress make it difficult to settle on the future course of treatment, but good practitioners rarely need to be over-optimistic.

There are some things which should quite definitely not happen in complementary treatment. On the practitioner's side, there should be no abuse of power. Your practitioner should not make any decisions or interfere in any way in your relationship, work or leisure activities. Practitioners may comment on how they see various things affecting your health, they may even suggest changes you could make to improve things, but any direct decision making and intervention is wrong. The same is true of treatment. It is not the practitioner's job to judge your healthcare decisions and it is certainly wrong if they demand you make changes.

> I had this woman coming to see me for massage, but her 'family therapist' insisted that she place herself exclusively in his care. Basically, he ordered her to stop coming here, though I am sure she didn't really want to.

The practitioner should also not make demands that clients adopt certain diet or lifestyle changes.

> His attitude was not 'I suggest you do ...' or 'I think it would be a good idea if you ...' He was all: 'Do this! Do that! I'll tell you what to do and you do it.' It was like a cult.

It is absolutely vital to keep in mind that it is you that has the health problem, it was your decision to consult the practitioner and it is the practitioner's role to offer skills and impartial advice to help you get yourself better. The purpose of treatment is not so that the practitioner can have a successful case history with which to boost his or her professional ego, neither is it for the practitioner to gain vicarious pleasure by experimenting with other people's lives.

Practitioners should also avoid laying 'guilt trips' on their clients. It is not the practitioner's job to give out moral judgements or to decide who should be ill or specify how someone ought to 'get their life together'. Health and morality are not easily combined: if you get ill, or if you fail to get better, this doesn't make you a bad person and practitioners who suggest otherwise should not be treating you or anyone else. (See also the section on 'Obstacles to healing' below).

If a practitioner adopts any position of power over a client, this should be seen as fatal to their relationship. It should also go without saying that sexual advances are completely out of the question.

On the other hand, there are also some behaviours that clients should avoid. Firstly, your practitioner may suggest you do certain things, for example, avoid coffee or practise a specific exercise. As has already been pointed out, you need not blankly nod 'Yes, Doctor' and blindly follow orders; you should discuss with your practitioner any doubts you have and mention anything you might find difficult. But once you have agreed on a plan of action, you must make your very best efforts to stick to it. If you fail, for whatever reason, you must be honest and tell your practitioner. Almost all medical practitioners, both complementary and conventional alike, have horror stories where clients have agreed to do something, failed to do it and then failed to mention that they have failed to do it. This not only makes treatment virtually impossible, it can actually be dangerous.

Another thing which you must be careful to avoid is taking advantage of your practitioner. Practitioners agree specified times to meet with clients and no matter how helpful, considerate and caring they might be during these treatment sessions, it is not their role to offer services at other times. You must not telephone at all times of the day and night to explain new symptoms or problems. Neither must you make demands on the practitioner in other ways.

> We agreed on 90 minute sessions for the massage, but each time, just as I was about to leave, Denise would burst into tears, look at me needily and say something designed to make me feel as though I should stay and chat and comfort her.

You may develop a wonderful relationship with your practitioner, but health professionals are not a replacement for friends and family and you should not treat them as such.

Obstacles to healing:
secondary gain and resisting change

One of the most thorny problems in complementary healthcare is when a practitioner suggests that a client is somehow preventing the healing process from taking place. It might sound strange that anyone would want to do this, and certainly many people are outraged and confused if the subject is brought up. But the fact that some people – perfectly sane, normal people – do things which block healing, is recognized by almost every health professional.

There are two reasons generally given as to why this might happen. The first is called 'secondary gain'. There are good and bad sides to all situations (winning the pools, after all, brings begging letters and accountants). In secondary gain, the positive sides to an illness or health problem are seen to interfere with recovery. The second reason given why individuals may block healing is that people tend to resist change and, put simply, becoming more healthy is a type of change.

Secondary gain

The typical cases of secondary gain discussed in the medical literature tend to involve people who either obtain some family advantage or manage to avoid some unpleasant situation as a result of being ill. If someone is unwell they might gain more attention from a spouse, receive a state benefit, avoid having to go to work, be able to spend more time with their children, avoid confronting marital or social problems or merely escape taking responsibility for themselves and others. Each of these is desirable. Some authors have noted that illness normally brings rewards such as care, attention and sympathy; many people say that being ill, and being able to stay home from school, is one of their best memories of childhood.

Resisting change

The idea of resisting change is often put like this: if an individual has a long-term problem, and if that problem influences many aspects of their lives, solving the problem will involve considerable personal change. And change is difficult. For example, Peter has had severe back pain for over two years. He has given up work and finds it hard to get out to the pub. His relationship with his wife has suffered and they no longer have sex. He has become very depressed and sits around the house doing little, becoming weaker through inactivity.

What part of Peter's life is unaffected by his pain problem? If Peter's condition were to improve, he would have to seek out employment, kick-start his social life and attempt a reconciliation with his wife. Each of these would be difficult and fraught with emotional pitfalls such as rejection. It is quite possible that some part of Peter would rather avoid these frightening changes and this may well compromise any attempts to overcome the pain problem.

It is also worth pointing out that secondary gain and resisting change can apply to families as well as to individuals. One family member might gain some benefit from another's illness, such as the woman who avoided confronting sexual problems with her husband by sleeping ('in case of emergency') with her asthmatic daughter, or the teenage boy who was able to do whatever he wanted because his parents were wrapped up in his brother's medical problems. Because the presence of a sick individual will affect the way any family operates, and because families tend to resist changes in the way they operate, improvements in a family member's condition can be resisted by the family. (See also the section on 'Family involvement' earlier in this chapter.)

Some people might think, 'That's ridiculous, no-one would put themselves through pain and suffering just to avoid an unpleasant situation or whatever'. The answer, of course, is that logically speaking, no-one would. But our minds, particularly our unconscious, do not necessarily work in logical ways. In fact, in many psychologists' understanding of the mind, the unconscious is partly defined by its lack of logic and rationality.

When you read about resisting change, or secondary gain, there is often an inclination to think of the individuals involved as stupid and ridiculous, as unpleasant manipulators. Consequently, it might be difficult for you to think how these problems might affect you personally, because no-one wants to be seen as stupid or manipulative. But it is worth remembering that such behaviours do not often take place deliberately; they are generally an unconscious and quite natural part of the healing process itself.

On the other hand, some people worry unduly that they are putting obstacles in their own path. Many individuals suffer agonies of guilt and self-doubt while they worry whether they are somehow to blame for their problems and whether the reason they are not getting better is simply that they can't get it together. Secondary gain seems to 'blame the victim' and some practitioners who have written about the subject have encouraged this with their 'I wash my hands of you' attitude. However, ideas such as obstacles to healing should really be seen not as a way of laying blame, nor as a way of rooting around looking for causes of problems, but as a way of maximizing the chances you have of getting the best from healthcare. Becoming aware that it is possible for individuals to compromise their own healing might prevent this circumstance happening to you.

Practitioners and 'obstacles to healing'

What happens if your practitioner implies that your progress is being impeded because somehow you 'want to be ill'? How do you know whether a practitioner has a case or whether he or she is just blaming their lack of success on your non-cooperation? Though there is no easy way out of this conundrum, it might be worth considering some of the following ideas.

If someone fails to benefit from healthcare, this does not necessarily mean that they are blocking their healing or that they somehow do not really want to get well. One reason to suspect that someone is resisting change is if they take certain actions or behave in certain ways which compromise the healing process. Such behaviours might include: forgetting to take pills at the appropriate time; being late for appointments or missing them entirely; failing to stick to diets; making excuses for not doing exercises set by the practitioner; constant indecision about treatment leading to a failure to do anything. Of course, everyone gets lazy or forgetful. But if you consistently act in ways which make getting better less likely, it is clear that you might have some resistance to change.

If your practitioner suggests that things are going slowly because you are blocking progress, discuss what specific actions you have taken which would bring about this end. Your practitioner might also discuss the subtle relationship between body and mind. The body and mind are, of course, interlinked, and there is little doubt that the mind can have a direct effect on the body without any physical action being taken. But what should you do if someone suggests that, without you realizing it, your own mind is preventing your body from getting well?

There are two ideas worth thinking about: firstly, self-understanding and, secondly, the role of the practitioner.

Given that it is possible for individuals, unconsciuosly, to block their healing, self-understanding must be seen as a crucial aspect of treatment. Some practitioners encourage their clients to ask: 'Why do I need this illness?' and there are a number of books which pose the same question. Perhaps a better way of putting this would be: 'What are all the advantages of my current situation? What are all the disadvantages?' Merely becoming aware of the hidden benefits of a situation you want to change can be a very important step. Similarly, asking: 'If my current situation improved, what would be the disadvantages and what would be the benefits?' might help to generate an awareness of the painful or difficult situations which an improvement might entail, and consequently, what might make healing more difficult.

Once you have made a conscious effort to understand which of your actions, if any, may have been interfering with treatment, and if you have tried to become more aware of what unconscious factors may be influencing your progress, then you have done your bit. Remember that the practitioner's job is to facilitate healing and that you may have paid him or her a lot of money to do this. If the practitioner implies, either directly or indirectly, that he or she cannot do much because somehow, you are not co-operating, ask the practitioner what he or she wants you to do. You might want to point out the ways in which you have already tried to understand your own obstacles to healing. Secondly, point out that good practitioners will not so easily be able to absolve themselves of responsibility. It is just no good for a practitioner to say: 'You are blocking your healing, that is why you are not getting better. I cannot help you 'til you pull yourself together'. A health professional worthy of the name will help you overcome such blocks. Solving problems in complementary healthcare is about co-operation between practitioner and client. This is as true for a secondary gain problem as for a back pain problem.

Perhaps most important of all, if some of the issues mentioned above do come up, you should never take it as an accusation of guilt, even if it is meant that way. Under no circumstances should you blame yourself or see yourself as a malingerer. Being ill can be painful, exhausting and deeply depressing. It is very likely that problems such as obstructing healing may in fact result from your condition. The energy that Peter, for example, has available to deal with problems like seeking work or patching things up with his wife, may have been drained by his pain problem. This vicious circle is experienced by many, many people and it is difficult to see how it could be wrong to experience something which so many others do when put in the same situation. And, as some workers have pointed out, resisting change is a perfectly normal human reaction.

Summary

It is important for users of complementary healthcare to play an active part in treatment. They must think hard about both themselves and their health problems and they must often decide between different healthcare options. Often, clients will be asked to make lifestyle and diet changes and be given exercises to do at home: in techniques such as yoga, tai chi or Alexander, daily practice is the most important part of treatment. If you play a 'sick role', and use your practitioner to fix you like you get the mechanic to fix your car, you are unlikely to make the most of complementary healthcare. Those individuals who benefit most tend to be those who take responsibility upon themselves and play an active and positive role in their treatment, particularly if they involve family or those around them.

It is uncommon for people to experience significant difficulties in complementary healthcare. One thing which can go wrong, however, is the relationship between practitioner and client. Practitioners should never take positions of power over clients; on the other hand, clients should avoid taking advantage of their practitioner.

One thorny problem is that people can sometimes block their own healing process. This can occur either because healing involves change and change is difficult or because there may be benefits in any situation and these will be lost if healing takes place. Such processes tend to occur without the individuals concerned being fully aware of them. However, practitioners should not accuse clients of doing this merely because they have been unsuccessful: it is necessary for both practitioner and client to work together to examine what actions the client may be taking which block the healing process and to think about the reasons why this might be so. Becoming aware that it is possible for individuals to compromise their own healing might prevent this circumstance from happening to you.

Part four

Appendices

Appendix A
Other disabilities

This appendix covers three areas: children with special needs; learning disabilities in older children and adults and physically disabling conditions which have not been mentioned in detail in the main text. It is worth pointing out that much of the book (for example, the section on 'How to choose a practitioner') remains relevant regardless of the disability or health problem which concerns you.

CHILDREN WITH SPECIAL NEEDS

The use of complementary therapies for children with special needs is a complex area and only the most brief and basic of introductions is possible here. See 'Further reading' for details of some books which touch on this subject.

Many disabled children suffer from a number of recurrent symptoms. These include: 'flu and respiratory infections; wheezing and coughing; bowel problems such as diarrhoea and constipation; 'glue ear'; sleep difficulties; poor circulation; vomiting and colic. Though it can often be helpful, orthodox drug treatment can sometimes actually exacerbate these problems or cause others. For example, antibiotics used to treat recurrent colds and 'flu often cause diarrhoea and they can increase a child's susceptibility to infection.

The advantage of complementary therapies is that they can sometimes treat symptoms without unwanted side-effects. Homoeopathy has proved to be a very popular treatment for many of the symptoms mentioned above: some parents have found that they can control, for example, their child's recurrent flu with homoeopathic medicine and they have been comforted by the thought that this is generally a harmless form of treatment. Other parents have noticed that their child has become stronger and less sickly after a course of homoeopathy: perhaps the most common phrase used by parents who have used complementary therapies for their children is: 'He's generally more healthy now'.

Therapies such as massage, aromatherapy, healing and reflexology appear to be effective at calming irritable and distracted children, often leading to improvements in sleeping patterns. Parents may find that children cease crying when they are placed on the treatment table and fall into a snooze while they are worked on. This calmness may last several days and, when hyperactivity and irritability return, they often do so with less intensity. Many parents have noticed a number of other benefits with these therapies: secondary symptoms, such as respiratory infections may improve and there may be an increase in general well-being, energy and alertness.

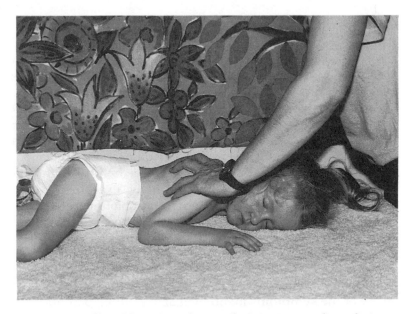

Figure Appendix 1 Massage and aromatherapy are popular techniques for work with children.

Some practitioners claim that sometimes, in addition to offering relief from symptoms, they are able to affect the intellectual and motor development of children with disabilities, particularly if treatment is started early enough. The claims of cranial osteopaths (see page 127) are particularly interesting in this respect. Cranial osteopaths believe that physical distortions of the nervous system, for example, an abnormal alignment of the bones of the skull, can impede development and that the correction of such distortions can often have important benefits. One common finding is that emotional and behavioural difficulties seem to subside after cranial osteopathy, but improvements in physical mobility are not unusual.

One acupuncturist who specializes in work with children has made a number of comments on Down's syndrome, and these can be seen as representative of the sort of claims that many complementary practitioners make about the treatment of disabled children.

> The severity of the signs can be reduced considerably. The dribbling, the inertia, the flaccid muscles largely disappear. The facial characteristics become less pronounced ... mentally they are still retarded ... but the indications are that some of the children at least will be able to fend for themselves when they grow up.

It is not entirely clear how claims such as this should be evaluated. Certainly, many disabled children have made remarkable progress after a course of complementary therapy; for others, however, benefits have not extended from relief of minor symptoms to an effect on motor and intellectual development. One thing which is apparent is that successful treatment takes a long period of time: weekly sessions for a year or so are not thought to be unusual.

The sections below give a little more information about specific conditions.

Autism

It seems that every autistic child can be reached in its own way: a number of orthodox and non-orthodox approaches have had success with a sub-group of autistic children and the complementary therapies are no different. Practitioners who work with touch (massage, osteopathy) or energy (healing, polarity) report moderate success with autistic children. The claims of the cranial osteopaths are occasionally more dramatic: at least one authority professes to be able to predict future autism purely on the basis of cranial bone structure.

Cerebral palsy

Acupuncture has been used with some success in children with cerebral palsy. Not only have there been a number of reports in the medical literature but the World Health Organization recognizes that acupuncture is an appropriate treatment for cerebral palsy. Acupuncture seems effective at improving muscle tone and decreasing spasm, and some practitioners say that it can help alertness and intelligence in those with learning disabilities. Practitioners of cranial osteopathy and Feldenkrais have also said that their therapies can be of benefit in cerebral palsy. See also discussions of complementary therapies for cerebral palsy in adults, throughout the book.

Hyperactivity

Where hyperactivity is not associated with another disability, food intolerance appears to be common (see the section on nutrition in Chapter 11) and an elimination diet is to be strongly recommended. Cranial osteopaths also say that they have had some success in treating hyperactivity.

Epilepsy

See page 259.

Muscular dystrophy

Many complementary practitioners have said that they have been able to improve quality of life and offer relief from symptoms in muscular dystrophy. One healer who had a child with muscular dystrophy said this of his son:

He had a high quality of life, he was basically happy. Throughout his life, the healing helped him cope psychologically. Near the end, it offered sleep and relief from pain.

Learning disability

Where learning disability is not associated with a specific condition (such as Down's syndrome) or with physical disability, complementary practitioners have reported some success in improving alertness, responsiveness and concentration in a proportion of clients. The three most commonly used therapies are homoeopathy, acupuncture and cranial osteopathy.

Down's syndrome

One of the main uses of complementary medicine in this condition is for the control of recurrent respiratory infections. Homoeopathy appears to be particularly successful and some parents have also tried milk-free and other food intolerance diets. Both cranial osteopaths and acupuncturists claim to be able to reduce physical symptoms (flaccid muscles, facial features, dribbling) if treatment is started early in life (see above). Some also say that intelligence might be improved in some cases. (See also 'Learning disability', below.)

LEARNING DISABILITY IN OLDER CHILDREN AND ADULTS

Yoga and relaxation techniques have been successfully used with groups of learning-disabled adults and children. Relaxation and concentration are aided and alertness can be increased. Maria Gunstone, who has considerable experience of teaching yoga to special needs groups, says that:

> Yoga can go a long way towards overcoming the frustration of not being able to communicate. The rewards [include] dramatically improved behaviour and physical co-ordination .... The pupils enjoy it so much, and have a tremendous sense of achievement when they can do the postures.

Massage and aromatherapy have been used extensively with those who have profound disabilities, especially at special schools and units. Touch is an especially effective means of communication and can be used to help foster relationships and overcome the defensiveness which is sometimes found in those with learning disabilities. Aromatherapy oils have also been used to create appropriate 'moods' in classrooms and as part of a 'sensory curriculum'. They also appear to be effective for minor complaints such as skin problems and respiratory infections.

PHYSICAL DISABILITIES NOT COVERED IN THE MAIN TEXT

The suggested therapies should be seen as general guidelines and pointers: remember that personal preference of therapy, and in particular, of practitioner, is of prime importance.

Sense impairment

People with visual impairments often have characteristic patterns of body tension associated with their disability. Where this has caused difficulties, massage, osteopathy and relaxation techniques such as yoga have been of benefit. Some blind people have poor body awareness: techniques such as the Alexander technique and Feldenkrais can help in this respect and some people have found that tai chi has helped them develop more flowing and confident movements. There are few health problems associated with deafness; however, a number of massage classes for mixed groups of hearing and non-hearing clients have explored the idea of communication through touch.

Asthma

It is difficult to make generalizations about complementary medicine and asthma because its causes, nature and responsiveness to treatment seem to vary enormously. Every individual will have a different experience: often, what works for one person with asthma will not work for another and, generally speaking, a number of different treatments need to be tried. Complementary healthcare rarely offers a total cure for asthma: in a typical successful case, attacks decline in frequency and severity and sometimes enable the gradual reduction of preventative medication such as steroids.

There is a great deal of scientific evidence on the effectiveness of complementary healthcare for asthma. Relaxation and meditation techniques, especially yoga, have been shown to be of some benefit in well-controlled trials and should be seen as strongly indicated. The literature on acupuncture and asthma is enormous, and highly contradictory: perhaps the most appropriate conclusion might be that acupuncture can help some people with asthma, but not others. Most homoeopaths are confident of treating asthma and there is at least some scientific justification for their claims. Intolerance to certain foods (see the section on nutrition in Chapter 11) appears to be implicated in at least some individuals, particularly those who have allergies, rashes etc. associated with their asthma. Finally, osteopaths and chiropractors say that asthmatic breathing can lead to problems of muscle tone and bone structure, something which of itself will exacerbate breathing difficulties.

Epilepsy

Like asthma, epilepsy seems to vary so much in cause, nature and responsiveness to treatment that it is difficult to make generalizations. In at least some people with epilepsy, seizures can be precipitated, or made more likely, by stress and anxiety. Because relaxation and meditation techniques can help reduce stress, as can therapies such as shiatsu, massage, healing and so on, it is perhaps not surprising that some individuals have reported reduced severity and frequency of seizures after using a relaxation discipline or therapy. Cranial osteopathy works with the nervous system and so might appear to be indicated in epilepsy, especially that precipitated by accident. Both acupuncture and herbal medicine have been shown to reduce frequency of seizures in laboratory animals. Acupuncture is particularly interesting because needling appears to cause the body to release a substance called GABA, the brain chemical which anti-epileptic medication simulates. Finally, there is evidence that particular foods can trigger seizures in at least some individuals, though the proportion concerned might be small (see section on nutrition in Chapter 11).

Cystic fibrosis

For recurrent respiratory infections, see 'Homoeopathy'. Therapies which calm and relax can be useful, especially those which involve the breath: yoga and meditation, relaxation and creative visualization. The role of nutrition is complex and might best be left to conventional physicians.

Haemophilia

The main use of complementary healthcare for people who have haemophilia is in the treatment of joint problems. Homoeopathy and acupuncture have been reported to improve pain and mobility in affected joints. See the sections in Chapters 6–12 on rheumatic conditions, though some material, such as that on nutrition, may not be relevant; see also the sections in these chapters dealing with chronic pain.

Repetitive strain injury (RSI)

This is a type of chronic pain associated wtih repeated actions such as typing or playing a musical instrument. It has also been reported in wheelchair users. Much of what has been written about chronic pain is applicable to RSI. The most essential element of treatment appears to be the breaking of the 'chronic pain syndrome' in which the depression and disability caused by pain and the dependence and frustration which result from trying to find a professional for a cure, of themselves contribute to the pain problem (see boxed section on pain at the beginning of Chapter 5). Self-help strategies such as yoga, tai chi and meditation seem particularly appropriate. Some workers have also emphasized the importance of de-medicalizing the problem, making less of a case of a damaged wrist or ligament, and more of an everyday difficulty caused by everyday factors such as stress, overwork and fatigue. Any reference to chronic pain in this book will generally be applicable for RSI.

Myalgic encephalomyelitis (ME)

Also known as post-viral fatigue syndrome, this is an unexplained condition which causes severe fatigue. It normally clears up with the passage of time, though some people remain affected for many years. Many complementary practitioners are confident of their ability to treat ME and certainly many of those with ME are relieved to have their problems taken seriously (some orthodox physicians believe that ME is an imaginary condition and that sufferers are malingering). In terms of complementary healthcare, there are a number of similarities between ME and multiple sclerosis – though the latter is generally more serious – so look under any sections referring to multiple sclerosis and see the discussion of disabling disease in Chapter 2 (page 26).

Diabetes

There is simply no replacement for insulin, where required. However, relaxation techniques such as yoga and meditation have been reported to reduce drug requirement in some people with maturity onset diabetes. Many complementary therapies (such as massage, aromatherapy, osteopathy) can improve poor blood circulation, a common consequence of diabetes. There have been reports of therapies such as reflexology and acupuncture being of help in other diabetes-related problems, such as neuropathy (the main symptom of which is a sensation of severe burning).

Eczema

Orally taken remedies seem indicated in eczema: recent trials have demonstrated the efficacy of Chinese herbal medicine; homoeopaths apparently have regular success with eczema and food intolerance (see the nutrition section in Chapter 11) appears implicated in some individuals. Acupuncturists have also claimed some success.

AIDS and cancer

These conditions are beyond the scope of this book. However, much of what is true for disabling diseases (e.g. multiple sclerosis) will hold for AIDS and cancer: see in particular the discussion in Chapter 2 (page 26). Bernie Siegel's books listed in 'Further reading' may be of interest, though see 'Do-it-yourself psychotherapy' in Chapter 13. *Surviving AIDS* by Michael Callen is also particularly recommended.

Appendix B
Funding complementary healthcare

Complementary healthcare is not widely available on the NHS and must usually be paid for privately. Unfortunately, one-to-one contact with a health professional does not come cheaply. The following examples of costs were compiled in mid-1992: prices may be cheaper outside London. A 'session' generally lasts an hour.

One session with an osteopath	£22
First session with an acupuncturist	£35
Subsequent sessions (½ hour)	£15
First session with a medically qualified homoeopath	£50
Subsequent sessions (15 mins – ½ hour)	£15
First session with a lay herbalist	£30
Subsequent sessions (½ hour)	£20
Individual tuition in the Alexander technique	£20
A full aromatherapy masage (1½ hours)	£35
One session of reflexology	£16
One yoga class through adult education	£1.50

Outcalls cost about another £5. You might also have to pay somewhere between £5 and £30 for a course of medicaments in herbal and homoeopathic medicine. It is easy to see how such costs can add up for a set of treatments or for regular sessions. However, most practitioners think that money should not be a barrier to treatment and many have sliding scales of fees or reserve a couple of appointments a week to give free of charge. If you have real financial difficulties, that is, if there is absolutely no possibility that could pay the full amount for treatment, you might be able to find a sympathetic practitioner who could offer you such a scheme.

On no account should you take unfair advantage of an offer of low cost treatment. Not only might you be preventing a more needy person from receiving treatment but you may put the practitioner off such schemes altogether. Most practitioners who no longer offer reduced fees do so because some clients have taken unfair advantage.

Though healthcare might appear expensive, it is also worth asking yourself how much your health is worth to you. For some reason, perhaps because we are so used to the NHS, many people become unreasonably miserly when it comes to paying for healthcare. It is not uncommon for someone whose health causes them problems every single day (a painful shoulder, an itchy skin rash) to balk at the thought of paying £150 or so for a set of sessions with a practitioner. When you think of the pain, aggravation and worry a health problem can cause, money put towards its alleviation might be considered money well spent.

Finally, if you encounter real problems funding complementary healthcare, there are a number of charitable trusts which give small grants to individuals in need though you normally require a social worker to write to a trust on your behalf. Charities such as RADAR can give you suitable advice on applying for grants.

Appendix C
Adverse reactions and contra-indications of complementary therapies

Adverse reactions from self-help or unregistered practitioners

Most of the adverse side-effects of complementary therapies found in the medical literature do not involve registered practitioners: this is one of the reasons why the use of the such professionals is recommmended. For example, a typical case of poisoning due to herbal medicine involved an 85 year old man who wandered into his garden, picked a plant and boiled up its leaves to make a tea. There do not seem to have been any instances of poisonings following a consultation with a herbalist registered by the National Institute of Medical Herbalists. In another well known case, an outbreak of hepatitis B was linked to the activities of an acupuncturist who had started up in practice despite having been refused registration by the appropriate body. Again, there have been no reported cases of insufficient needle sterilization amongst registered practitioners of acupuncture. Each of the aromatherapy oils has a variety of contraindications, the most common of which are epilepsy and skin conditions. This is one of the reasons why consulting a competent practitioner of aromatherapy is so important.

Adverse effects have been reported for individuals trying unusual complementary therapies (those not mentioned in this book) particularly where a practitioner has suggested a diet. But self-help diets have also caused problems: there has been a report of a young couple who decided to try macro-biotics, bought a book and strictly followed its recommendations until the woman died of malnutrition. Overdoses on nutritional supplements are quite common where individuals have used off-the-shelf vitamin pills without professional guidance.

Less serious side-effects are also common with unregistered practitioners. One woman reported that she was in fairly severe pain for a whole day following a massage. Who had given her the massage? A friend who had been on a weekend class. Another individual reported having woken up with an agonizing headache following a reflexology treatment from someone yet to complete a course in the technique. You can get a gentle, relaxing back or foot rub from just about anyone, but someone who is not fully trained should not try anything 'therapeutic', especially on someone who has a disability or a serious health condition.

In summary, if you wish to reduce your chances of an adverse reaction from complementary medicine, use registered practitioners, avoid unusual therapies and be careful with self-help.

Minor side-effects of complementary therapies

Mild adverse reactions are a relatively common feature of complementary therapies. The overwhelming majority follow the first treatment, and are often taken as a positive sign by practitioners. For example, a bout of diarrhoea and sweating brought on by reflexology, may be seen as a sign that the body's elimination systems have been stimulated by the treatment.

Mild reactions common to all complementary therapies include drowsiness and light headedness. A common feeling is 'I can't keep myself upright'. The muscles the body uses to support itself lose their tone and this may even cause a transient bout of clumsiness. This is not actually an unpleasant experience: it feels little different from waking up after a particularly long and restful lie-in. Also in common with the lie-in there may be slight feeling of malaise (i.e. unease or sickness) after a treatment session. These feelings soon pass and if you have arranged time to wind down after your session, as is suggested in Chapter 14, these effects should cause few problems.

Acupuncture, shiatsu and reflexology have a similar set of mild side-effects. Headache is common after the first treatment; longer lasting effects may include increased sweating and urination, diarrhoea, flatulence and, rarely, even skin irritation or spots. Practitioners believe that these effects are due to increased activity of the elimination systems of the body.

As with homoeopathy, herbal medicine and dietary therapy, aggravation reactions may also occur. These involve a slight worsening of symptoms and are taken as a positive sign that healing is taking place. Though aggravation reactions are generally harmless, care must be taken in diseases such as asthma or cystic fibrosis where any exacerbations could have serious consequences. You may also find that symptoms change and move about in unusual ways: for example, you start getting arthritis in your hands just as your shoulder pains clear up, or you might experience a recurrence of childhood eczema. Again, these reactions are generally harmless and indicate that healing is going well. Osteopathy and chiropractic may also occasionally bring about reactions like sweating or diarrhoea. Much more common, however, is a feeling of diffuse pain, not unlike bruising, which lasts perhaps 6–8 hours after treatment. This normally occurs after the first session and you will rarely have to experience it twice. Some people complain of general aches and pains lasting for several days; again, these are harmless and rarely recur. Very occasionally, manipulation causes more distressing effects such as feelings of cold, nausea, fainting or palpitations and there may even be a recurrence of the original pain or new pains in the pelvis or abdomen. Such reactions should be reported to the practitioner.

Some individuals report muscle pain on the day following a session of Alexander technique or Feldenkrais. This may last several days and is often accompanied by fatigue and a feeling of 'I don't know how my body is', almost a sort of clumsiness. Practitioners claim that this is a result of real changes taking place in the client's body and in the way in which he or she uses it.

Finally if, after treatment, anything which happens to your body and worries or concerns you, tell your practitioner. He or she may well be able to allay any fears or take appropriate action if anything serious has happened. If you are still concerned, inform your GP.

Serious adverse reactions from complementary medicine

Fortunately, these are rare. Complications of acupuncture which have been reported include pneumothorax (collapse of a lung), needles found in various body cavities and even heart failure. Each of these is attributable to bad technique and must be seen as exceptionally unlikely to happen to an individual consulting a registered acupuncturist in the UK.

Serious adverse reactions to osteopathy and chiropractic may occur if manipulation to a weakened joint damages surrounding nerves or blood vessels. Stroke has been reported as a consequence of manipulation to the cervical spine (the bones of the neck) and damage to the spinal cord itself is not unknown. However, such side-effects are extremely rare: one study estimates that out of every 100 000 cervical manipulations (which, of course, do not happen every treatment) only two will result in some sort of neurological complication and just 0.1 will result in some major event such as spinal cord damage. It is likely that improved knowledge and technique will further reduce such occurrences.

Compare such figures with the estimate that, in the USA over 60 000 people die annually from side-effects of medicines and over 60% of hospitalized patients have adverse drug reactions. In summary, you are highly unlikely to have any serious side-effects as a result of complementary treatment.

Contraindications to complementary medicine

A contraindication is a sign that it might be dangerous to use a particular drug or medical technique. For example, cortisone skin cream is contraindicated if the skin is broken or infected, such as in acne, burns or cold sores. You musn't use cortisone cream on broken or infected skin because there is a chance of the drug getting into the bloodstream and causing complications.

Most practitioners of complementary healthcare are well versed in the contraindications to their therapies. In general, complementary therapies are contraindicated during acute stages or exacerbations of disease. If, say, you have a flare up of rheumatoid arthritis, any treatment whch involves touch or movement should be avoided; osteopaths, for example, are taught not to manipulate inflamed joints. Similarly, if you catch 'flu or some serious infection, most complementary therapies should be avoided, though obviously homoeopathy and herbal medicine are exceptions to this.

The other main contraindications are listed in various places throughout this book. They are:

- When medical attention is urgently required, for example, after an accident, and where complementary healthcare would be time consuming.
- Various aromatherapy oils for people with epilepsy or skin conditions (see the first paragraph in this appendix – page 266).
- The relaxation technique known as 'sequential muscle holding' for some people with stroke, multiple sclerosis and brain injuries (see meditation, relaxation and creative visualization). This technique must also be used with some care for people with joint problems.
- Some yoga and tai chi positions for people with joint problems (see yoga and tai chi).
- Some osteopathic and chiropractic manipulations for people with advanced joint disease.
- Massage and reflexology where skin is broken or infected (e.g. in burns or fungal infection).
- A number of different techniques are contraindicated in pregnancy. In particular, care must be exercised with aromatherapy, herbal medicine, and nutritional therapy.
- You should avoid combining complementary and conventional medicine into a single treatment. For example, a man who used yoga breathing to increase the effectiveness of his asthma inhaler ended up in hospital.

Appendix D
Information for disability professionals considering using complementary therapies in a disability setting

A number of physiotherapists, key workers and other disability professionals have expressed an interest in the idea of incorporating complementary therapies into the work at their unit. Here are a number of issues worth considering.

Competence

How will the competence of complementary practitioners be assessed? Will indemnity insurance be affected? What if something goes wrong?

Training

Will the complementary practitioners receive any special training? Few practitioners have a robust understanding of the medical and social aspects of disability; moreover, most have had little experience of a working situation in which they must work as part of a team and take instructions from a manager. Some practitioners also have difficulties with assessment procedures.

Evaluation

Will the complementary therapies be evaluated? If so, how?

Practice

How will clients come to receive complementary healthcare? Should they choose a practitioner/therapy at will or should this be guided in some way?

Liaison

Complementary therapies appear to work most effectively when they are used as an integral part of a programme of care at a unit, rather than just as a supplementary add-on. At some units, practitioners have sometimes kept themselves to themselves, working quietly in a closed-off room and leaving at the end of the day without significant contact with workers. At other units, practitioners have been involved in discussions about users and have shared their observations; liason between complementary practitioners and other workers has been maximized and the skills and strengths of each group have been utilized in the most appropriate way. (See also the discussion on page 9.)

Power relations

Complementary practitioners should not be treated as 'junior partners': all health professionals co-operating on the care of an individual should be accorded equal status – and equal responsibilities. Complementary practitioners should not be allowed to think themselves 'above' meetings, evaluations, reports and other more mundane elements of disability work.

Finance

It is recommended that complementary practitioners should be paid: a volunteer status does not encourage optimal liaison or equitable power relations.

Mutual understanding

Complementary practitioners may hold a very different philosophy of health care to other workers. There should be an attempt on both sides to understand and allow for differences in beliefs, aims and methods.

Appendix E
Information for complementary practitioners interested in working with disabled people

Working with disabled people does not present any great and mysterious challenges to a complementary practitioner. However, there may be a number of things practitioners might like to think about before working with a disabled client, especially if they do so in a setting such as a day centre or rehabilitation unit.

Access

Would it be possible for a physically disabled person to reach the treatment room? How could access be improved? What about outcalls?

Social aspects of disability

Many disabled people tend to play down the medical aspects of disability. The reasons for this are not hard to fathom: disabled people are often treated as a function of their condition and endure extreme prejudice as a result. For example, those with physical disbilities are often deemed incapable of intellectual effort, even to the point of making trivial decisions ('Does he take sugar?'). Disabled people point out that popular fiction often associates moral weakness with physical stigma (Dr Strangelove, Captain Hook) and that the media rarely portrays disabled people outside the role of 'heroes' or 'cabbages'. Disabled people are excluded from many things which able-bodied people take for granted. Public transport is almost always inaccessible for people in wheelchairs; likewise, physical barriers such as steps and narrow doors often prevent those with disabilities from using shops, cinemas, libraries, restaurants and hotels. Employment opportunities are often restricted, by inaccessible buildings and by the prejudice of employers.

Empowerment

Many disabled people feel disempowered, particularly in medical contexts. It is worth considering whether the health techniques you use give power to the client or are just one more health technique, one more thing done to them. Moreover, it is important to ensure that clients are given the maximum possible choice over treatment decisions. For example, some practitioners who work in day centres have asked potential clients direct to their faces if they wanted treatment. It would be embarrassing and difficult for most people to refuse in such a situation, even more so for someone used to being at the mercy of other people's decisions. A better situation would be to allow the individuals concerned to make up their mind in another room and relay their decision through a third party if necessary.

Liaison

A number of different professionals may liaise on the care of a person with a disability. These may include a social worker, a physiotherapist, an occupational therapist, a consultant, a GP, 'key workers', and workers at day centres and other units. It is important for complementary practitioners to maintain effective relations with these individuals.

Practice

Complementary practitioners may be taught generalizations about the body which may no longer hold true when disability is involved.

Personal issues

It is important for complementary practitioners working with disabled people to consider their reasons and aims. Some workers have found it emotionally difficult to work with clients who do not improve as rapidly or dramatically as others; other workers have been surprised that disabled people have found their attitudes to be deeply patronizing. It can sometimes be a help to contact other practitioners who have worked with disabled people for support and advice.

Appendix F
Other organizations including those outside the UK

Research Council for Complementary Medicine (RCCM)
60 Great Ormond Street, London WC1N 3JF. Tel 071-833 8897.
   Promotes rigorous research into complementary medicine.
   The RCCM also runs a literature searching service for
   information on medical research.

Council for Complementary and Alternative Medicine (CCAM)
179 Gloucester Place, London NW1 6DX. Tel 071-724 9103.
   Umbrella body for acupuncture, herbal medicine, homoeopathy and osteopathy. However, not all practitioners
   of these therapies are registered with CCAM.

Institute for Complementary Medicine
Tavern Quay, London SE16 Postal Address: PO Box 194,
   London SE16 1QZ. Tel 071-237 5165.
   Information on complementary medicine. Administers the
   British Register of complementary practitioners (see page
   12) and can refer enquirers to competent therapists. Also,
   a useful source of information on training and courses.
   Enclose a large SAE when contacting the Institute for
   Complementary Medicine.

SCOPE
160 Fernhead Road, London W9 3EL.
   SCOPE aims to promote the health and independence of
people with severe disabilities by the use of complementary therapies.

Multiple Sclerosis Healing Trust
c/o Ray Jordan, 64 Holly Road, Oldbury, Warley,
West Midlands B68 0AT.
Treatment of people who have multiple sclerosis using
complementary therapies, some of which fall at the more
unusual end of the spectrum.

Health Information Service
Tel 0438 314333, ext 520.

Help for Health
Tel 0962 849100.

Both organizations can help put you in touch with support
groups for a variety of conditions.

Foreign organizations

If you have trouble locating a suitable practitioner outside of
the UK, try contacting one of the British organizations listed
in Chapter 5.

American Academy of Osteopathy
1127 Mount Vernon Road, PO Box 750, Newark, Ohio
43058-0750, USA.

Australian Council on Chiropractic and Osteopathic Education
941 Nepean Highway, Mornington, Victoria 3931, Australia.

New Zealand Register of Osteopaths
PO BOX 11–853, Wellington 1, New Zealand.

International Society for Clinical and Experimental Hypnosis
PO BOX 298, Belmead, New Jersey 08502, USA.

American College of Nutrition
722 Robert E Lee Drive, Wilmington, North Carolina 20927,
USA.

American Institute of Homoeopathy
1500 Massachusetts Avenue NW, Washington DC 20005, USA.

Canadian Society of Homoeopathy
PO Box 4333, Station East, Ottawa, Canada K15 5B3.

North American Society of Homoeopaths
4712 Aldrich Avenue, Minneapolis 55409, USA.

Australian Institute of Homoeopathy
21 Bulah Close, Berowra Heights, Sydney, NSW 2082, Australia.

New Zealand Homoeopathic Society
PO Box, 67095, Mt Eden, Auckland, New Zealand.

New Zealand Institute of Classical Homoeopathy
24 Westhaven Drive, Tawa, Wellington, New Zealand.

Australian Society of Teachers of the Alexander Technique
PO Box 529, Milsons Point, Sydney 2061, New South Wales,
  Australia.

Canadian Society of Teachers of the Alexander Technique
460 Palmerston Boulevard, Toronto, Ontario, P7A 4A2.

**North American Society of Teachers of the Alexander
  Technique**
PO Box 806, Ansonia Station, New York, NY 10023-0806, USA.

American Association of Acupuncture and Oriental Medicine
National Acupuncture Headquarters, 1424 16th Street NW,
  Suite 501, Washington DC 20036, USA.

Acupuncture Ethics and Standards Organization
PO BOX 84, Merrylands, NSW 2160, Australia.

New Zealand Register of Acupuncturists
PO BOX 9950, Wellington 1, New Zealand.

National Herbalists Association of Australia
247–9 Kingsgrove Road, Kingsgrove, SA 2208.

American Herb Association
PO Box 353, Rescue, California 96672, USA.

Further reading

Listed below are a few select books on complementary healthcare. Some may no longer be available in print. Your practitioner might be able to give you some more suggestions, as might organizations of complementary medicine such as the Society of Homoeopaths. In general you should choose healthcare books using similar criteria to those you might use to decide on a practitioner (see page 49). For example, you should avoid books which offer guarantees of successful results or which promise to make your whole life perfect. Another hint is to avoid books which feature letters from grateful clients. For example, you should steer well clear if the cover blurb includes: '"Since I went on your diet, I've been pain free! I can't thank you enough!" – Mrs F, Leeds'.

INTRODUCTIONS TO THERAPIES FOR PROSPECTIVE CLIENTS

Korle, Hellmut (1988) *Hypnosis and Hypnotherapy: A Patients' Guide*. Thorsons.
Grove-Stephenson, Ian and Quilliam, Susan (1990) *The Best Counselling Guide*. Thorsons.
McIntyre, Anne (1987) *Herbal Medicine*. Optima.
Moore, Susan (1987) *A Guide to Chiropractic*. Hamlyn.
Sandler, Stephen (1987) *A Guide to Osteopathy*. Hamlyn.
Stevens, Chris (1987) *Alexander Technique*. Optima.
Worsley, J.R. (1988) *Acupuncture: Is it for you?* Element.

SELF-HELP GUIDES

Brosnan, Barbara (1986) *Yoga for Handicapped People*. Human Horizons.
Benson, Herbert (1988) *The Relaxation Response*. Collins.

280 *Further reading*

Catalano, Ellen Mohr (1987) *The Chronic Pain Control Workbook.* New Harbinger Publications.
Downing, George (1972) *The Massage Book.* Penguin.
Feldenkrais, Moshe (1981) *Awareness Through Movement.* Penguin.
Graham, Judy (1987) *Multiple Sclerosis: A Self-help Guide to its Management.* Thorsons.
Graham, Margaret (1988) *Keep Moving, Keep Young: Gentle Yoga Exercises for the Elderly.* Unwin Hyman.
Kent, Howard (1985) *Yoga for the Disabled: A Practical Self-help Guide.* Thorsons.
Long, Barry (1986) *Meditation: A Foundation Course.* Barry Long Foundation.
Mitchell, Laura (1987) *Simple Relaxation.* John Murray.
Worwood, Valerie Ann (1990) *The Fragrant Pharmacy* (a book on aromatherapy). Macmillan.

SELF-HELP GUIDES TO NUTRITION AND DIET

ARMS (1986) *Why a Diet Rich in Essential Fatty Acid?* ARMS.
Brostoff, Jonathan and Gamlin, Linda (1989) *The Complete Guide to Food Allergy and Intolerance.* Bloomsbury.
Fitzgerald, Gerlaldine and Briscoe, Fennella (1988) *Multiple Sclerosis Cookbook.* Thorsons.
Workman, E., Alun Jones, V. and Hunter, J. (1986) *The Food Intolerance Diet Book.* Martin Dunitz.

GENERAL INTEREST

Boston Women's Health Book Collective (1989) *The New Our Bodies, Our Selves: A Book by, for and about Women.* Penguin.
Callen, Michael (1991) *Surviving AIDS.* Harper Perennial.
Cousins, Norman (1981) *Anatomy of an Illness as Perceived by the Patient.* Bantam.
Forsythe, Elizabeth (1988) *Multiple Sclerosis: Exploring Sickness and Health.* Faber & Faber.
Siegel, Bernie S. (1986) *Love, Medicine and Miracles.* Century-Hutchinson Rider.
Siegel, Bernie S. (1990) *Peace, Love and Healing.* Century-Hutchinson Rider.
Werbach, Melvyn R. (1986) *Third Line Medicine.* Arkana.

COMPLEMENTARY HEALTHCARE AND OTHER DISABILITIES

Sanderson, Helen and Harrison, Jane with Shirley Price (1991) *Aromatherapy and Massage for People with Learning Difficulties*. Hands On Publishing.

Vickers, Andrew (in press) *Health Options: Complementary medicine for children with disabilities*. Element Books.

Bibliography

To avoid breaking the flow of the text, footnotes and referencing were not used in the main text of this book. A variety of papers from the medical literature are listed below: all studies and reports mentioned in the text can be located in this bibliography, though some will be contained in reviews and monographs.

There follows three lists of topics: disabilities, therapies and miscellaneous. The numbers after each topic refer to the Reference list which starts on page 285.

Disabilities

Abbreviations

ACUP = Acupuncture; AROMA = Aromatherapy; CNSL = Counselling; EMG = Biofeedback; HEAL = Healing; HERB = Herbal Medicine; HOM = Homoeopathy; HYPN = Hypnotherapy; MAN = Osteopathy and chiropractic; NUTR = Nutritional therapy; INTOL = Food intolerance diet; EFA = Fats in the diet; SUPPL = Vitamin and mineral supplements; RLX = Relaxation techniques/meditation; ROLF = Rolfing; SHIA = Shiatsu/acupressure; SLF = Self-help; TAI = Tai chi; YOGA = Yoga.

Amputation: HYPN 1; ACUP 2–3
Asthma: ACUP 5–9; RLX 10, 12, 223; HYPN 11, 13; YOGA 14–7; HOM 18; INTOL 19–21; MAN 22, 83
Cerebral injury: (see also *Stroke*) ACUP 3, 282; RLX 163; SHIA 282
Cerebral palsy: ROLF 24; RLX 25, 74; ACUP 26–29, 282; MAN 30; SHIA 282

Therapies

Citations marked with an asterisk refer to scientific trials
or laboratory studies which touch on the question of efficacy, i.e. whether complementary therapies can be said to
work.

Other topics

Adverse effects of complementary healthcare: 83, 181–5
Adverse effects of conventional medicine: 187
Stress and the role of the mind in disease: 81, 187–8, 210, 214,
216–20, 223, 231–43, 245–51, 269–70

REFERENCES

Abbreviations

Acupunct = Acupuncture; *Am* = American; *Ann* = Annals;
Arch = Archives: *Arth* = Arthritis; *Assoc* = Association;
Aust = Australia; *Behav* = Behaviour/behavioral; *Br* = British;
Bull = Bulletin; *Can* = Canadian; *Chin* = Chinese; *Chirop* =
Chriopractic; *Chron* = Chronic; *Clin* = Clinical; *Complement*
= Complementary; *Dev* = Developmental; *Diet* = Dietetic;
Dis = Disease; *Electrotherap* = Electrotherapeutics; *Ethno-
pharmacol* = Ethnopharmacology; *Exp* = Experimental; *Hom* =
Homoeopathy; *Immun* = Immunology; *Int* = International;
Intern = Internal; *J* = Journal; *Med* = Medicine/medical;
Neurol = Neurology; *Nurs* = Nursing; *Occup* = Occupational;
Osteo = Osteopathy; *Paediatr* = Paediatric; *Phys* = Physical;
Physiol = Physiology; *Pract* = practitioner; *Psychiat* =
Psychiatric/psychiatry; *Psychol* = Psychological/psychology;
Psychosom = Psychosomatic; *R* =Royal; *Rehab* = Rehabilitation;
Res = Research; *Rev* = Review; *Rheum* = Rheumatic/
rheumatism; *Rheumatol* = Rheumatology; *Scand* = Scan-
dinavian; *Sci* = Science/sciences; *Semin* = Seminars; *Soc* =
Social; *Ther* = Therapy; *Tradit* = Traditional; *Urol* = Urology

{TR} = Clinical trial; {LAB} = Laboratory/animal experiment;
{CN} = Case Report(s) or retrospective observations of prac-
titioner; {BB} = Includes useful bibliographic information; {RV}
= Review; {M} = Monograph

1. Minichello, W.E. (1987) Treatment of hyperhidrosis of
   amputation site with hypnosis and suggestions involving
   classical conditioning. *Int J Psychosom*, 34(4): 7–8. {CN}
2. Sidlow, C.J., Frankel, S.L., Chiros, P.G., Hamilton, V.
   (1989) Electroacupuncture therapy for stump neuroma pain:
   a case report. *J Am Podiatric Med Assoc*, 79(1): 31–4. {CN}

3. Freed, S. (1989) Acupuncture as therapy of traumatic affective disorders and of phantom limb pain syndrome. *Acupunct Electrotherap Res*, 14(2): 121–9. {CN}

4. Owens, M.K. and Ehrenreich, D. (1991) Literature review of nonpharmacologic methods for the treatment of chronic pain. *Holistic Nurs Pract*, 6(1): 24–31. {RV}

5. Aldridge, D. and Pietroni, P.C. (1987) Clinical assessment of acupuncture in asthma therapy: discussion paper. *J R Soc Med*, 80(4): 222–4. {RV}

6. Kleijnen, J., ter Riet, G. and Knipschild, P. (1991) Acupuncture and asthma: a review of controlled trials *Thorax* 46(11): 799–802. {RV} {BB}

7. Maharaj, K., Tandon, M.D. and Soh, P.F.T. (1989) Comparison of real and placebo acupuncture for histamine induced asthma. *Chest*, 96(1): 102–5. {TR}

8. Fung, K.P., Chow, O.K. and So, S.Y., (1986) Attenuation of exercise induced asthma. *Lancet*, 2: 1419–21. {TR}

9. Jobst, K.M. *et al.* (1986) Controlled trial of acupuncture for disabling breathlessness. *Lancet*, 2: 1416   18. {TR}

10. Kinsman, R.A. *et al.* (1980) Anxiety reduction in asthma: four catches to general application. *Psychosom Med*, 42; 397–405. {RV}

11. Ewer, T.C. and Stewart, D.E. (1986) Improvement of bronchial hyper-responsiveness in patients with moderate asthma after treatment with a hypnotic technique: a randomised controlled trial. *Br Med J (Clin Res)*, 293(6555): 1129–32. {TR}

12. Lehrer, P.M. (1986) Relaxation decreases large airway but not small airway asthma. *J Psychosom Res*, 30(1): 13–25. {TR}

13. Morrison, J.C. (1988) Chronic asthma and improvement with relaxation induced by hypnotherapy. *J R Soc Med*, 81(12): 701–4. {TR}

14. Nagarathna, R. and Nagendra, H.R. (1985) Yoga for bronchial asthma: a controlled study. *Br Med J (Clin Res)*, 291(6502): 1077–9. {TR}

15. Nagarathna, R. and Nagendra, N.R. (1986) A controlled approach of yoga therapy for bronchial asthma: a 3–54 month prospective study. *J Asthma*, 23(3): 123–7. {TR}

16. Singh, V., Wisniewski, A., Britton, J. and Tattersfield, A. (1990) Effect of yoga breathing exercises (pranayama)

on airway reactivity in subjects with asthma. *Lancet*, 335: 1381–3. {TR}

17. Jain, S.C. *et al.* (1991) Effect of yoga training on exercise tolerance in adolescents with childhood asthma. *J Asthma*, 28(6): 437–42. {RV}.

18. Reilly, D.T., Taylor, M.A., Campbell, J. *et al.* (1990) Is homoeopathy a placebo response? A controlled trial of homoeopathic immunotherapy (HIT) in atopic asthma (abstract). *Proceedings of the 45th Congress of the Liga Medicorum Homoeopathica Internationalis.* {TR}

19. Lindahl, O. *et al.* (1985) Vegan diet regimen with reduced medication in the treatment of bronchial asthma. *J Asthma*, 22(1): 45–55. {TR}

20. Hoj, L. (1981) A double blind controlled trial of elemental diet for severe perennial asthma. *Allergy*, 36: 257–62. {TR}

21. Wraith, D.G. (1987) Asthma. In *Food Allergy and Intolerance*, Brostoff, J. and Challacombe, S.J. (eds.) Baillière Tindall, Eastbourne. {RV}{BB}

22. Renaud, C.I. and Pichette, D. (1990) Chiropractic management of bronchial asthma: a literature review. *J Chiropractic*, 27(12): 25–6. {RV}

23. Master, F.J. (1988) An homoeopathic approach to the neurology of the hereditary ataxias. *Proceedings of the 43rd Congress of the International Homoeopathic Medical League*: 86–90. {CN}

24. Perry, J., Jones, M.H. and Thomas, L. (1981) Functional evaluation of rolfing in cerebral palsy. *Dev Med Child Neurol*, 23: 717–29. {TR}

25. O'Donoghue, P. (1988) Relaxation in cerebral palsy. *Dev Med Child Neurol*, 30(1): 115–25. {TR}

26. Filipowicz, W.A. (1991) The application of modern acupuncture techiques and methods on children with cerebral palsy. *Am J Acup*, 19(1): 5–10. {TR}

27. Sammer, G. *et al.* (1981) Acupuncture for the relief of painful muscular spasm in dystonic cerebral palsy. *Dev Med Child Neurol*, 23(4): 544–5. {CN}

28. Semenova, K.A. (1985) [Clinico-biochemical indicators of the effectiveness of acupuncture in children with cerebral palsy (spastic diplegia) during the first two years of life]. *Paediatrica*, 10: 58–60. [Russian]. {CN}

288 Bibliography

29. Bingpei, S. *et al*. (1992) A clinical study on acupuncture treatment of paediatric cerebral palsy. *J Tradit Chin Med*, 12(1): 45–51. {CN}
30. Fryman, V. (1966) Relation of disturbances of craniosacral mechanisms to symptomatology of the new born. *J Am Osteo Assoc*, 65: 1059–1072. {CN}
31. Vickers, A. (1993) Homoeopathy and Disability. *Br Hom J*, 82: 53–7. {RV}
32. Evans, F.J. (1989) Hypnosis and chronic pain: two contrasting case studies. *Clin J. Pain*, 5(2): 169–76. {CN}
33. Hawkins, R. (1988) The role of hypnotherapy in the pain clinic. *Aust J Clin Exp Hypn*, 16(1): 23–30. {CN}
34. Colosimo, C.P. (1989) The use of self hypnosis in the mangement of chronic pain. *Hypnos*, 16(3): 122–6. {CN}
35. James, F.R., Large, R.G. and Bealem, I.L. (1989) Self-hypnosis in chronic pain: A multiple baseline study of five highly hypnotisable subjects. *Clin J Pain*, 5(2): 161–8. {TR}
36. Kabat-Zinn, J., Lipworth, L. and Burney, R. (1985) The clinical use of mindfulness meditation for self-regulation of chronic pain. *J Behav Med* , 8(2): 163–90. {TR}
37. Linton, S.J. (1986) Behavioral remediation of chronic pain: a status report. *Pain*, 24(2): 125–4. {RV}
38. Philips, H.C. (1988) Changing chronic pain experience. *Pain*, 32(2): 165–72. {TR}
39. Shaw, L. and Ehrlich, A. (1987) Relaxation training as a treatment for chronic pain caused by ulcerative colitis. *Pain*, 29(3): 287–93. {RV}
40. Nespar, K. (1991) Pain management and yoga. *Int J Psychosom*, 38(1–4): 76–81. {RV}{BB}
41. Turner, J.A. (1982) Comparison of group progressive-relaxation training and cognitive behavioral group therapy for chronic low back pain. *J Consult Clin Psychol*, 50: 757–65. {TR}
42. Strong, J. (1991) Relaxation training and chronic pain. *Br J Occup Ther*, 47(3): 743–61. {TR}
43. Richardson, P.H. and Vincent, C.A. (1986) Acupuncture for the treatment of pain: a review of evaluative research. *Pain*, 24: 15–40. {RV}{BB}
44. Peng, A.T.C., Behar, S. and Yue, S.J. (1987) Long term therapeutic effects of electro-acupuncture for chronic neck

and shoulder pain – a double blind study. *Acup Electrotherap Res*, 12: 37–44. {TR}

45. Patel, M., Gutzwiller, F., Paccaud, F. and Marazzi, A. (1989) A meta-analysis of acupuncture for chronic pain. *Int J Epidemiol*, 18(4): 900–6. {RV}

46. Riet ter, G., Kleijnen, J. and Knipschild, P. (1990) Acupuncture and chronic pain: a criteria based meta-analysis. *J Clin Epidemiol*, 43: 1191–9. {RV}{BB}

47. Junnila, S.Y. (1987) Long-term treatment of chronic pain with acupuncture: part I. *Acup Electrotherap Res*, 12(1): 23–36. {TR}

48. Junnila, S.Y. (1987) Long-term treatment of chronic pain with acupuncture: part II. *Acup Electrotherap Res*, 12(1): 125–38. {TR}

49. Berlin, J., Erdman, W. and David, E. (1989) Psychosomatic correlations in chronic pain patients using electroacupuncture. *Am J Chin Med*, 17(1–2): 85–7. {CN}

50. Fisher, K. (1988) Early experiences of a multidisciplinary pain management programme. *Holistic Med*, 3(1): 47–56. {CN}

51. Wright, S.M. (1987) Use of therapeutic touch in the management of pain. *Nurs Clin North Amer*, 2(3): 705–14. {CN}

52. Jack, R.A. (1988) Anecdotal but significant. *Br Hom J*, 77(1): 4–11. {CN}

53. Shanmugasundaram, E.R., Mohammed Akbar, G.K. and Radha Shanmugasundaram, K. (1991) Brahmighritham: an Ayurvedic herbal formula for the control of epilepsy. *J Ethnopharmacol*, 33(3): 269–76. {LAB}

54. Sugaya, E., Ishige, A., Sekiguchi, K., Iiszuka, S., Sugimotoo, A., Yuzurihara, M. and Hosoya, E. (1988) Inhibitory effect of a mixture of herbal drugs (TJ-960, SK) on pentylenetrazol induced convulsions in El mice. *Epilepsy Res*, 2(5): 337–9. {LAB}

55. Li, W. *et al.* (1989) Double-blind crossover controlled study on antiepilepsirine. *Chin Med J*, 102(2): 79–85. {TR}

56. Tozzo, C.A., Elfner, L.F. and May, J.G. (1988) EEG biofeedback and relaxation training in the control of epileptic seizures. *Int J Psychophysiol*, 6(3): 185–94. {TR}

57. Shi, Z. *et al.* (1987) The efficacy of electro-acupuncture on 98 cases of epilepsy. *J Tradit Chin Med*, 7(1): 21–2. {TR}

58. Wu, D. (1988) Suppression of epileptic seizures with acupuncture: efficacy, mechanism and perspective. *Am J Acupunct*, 16(2): 113–7. {LAB}

59. Crayton, J.W., Stoe, T. and Stem, G. (1981) Epilepsy precipitated by food sensitivity: report of a case with double-blind placebo controlled assessment. *Clin Electro-encephalography*, 12: 192–8. {CN}

60. Bell, I.R. (1987) Effects of food allergy on the central nervous system. In *Food Allergy and Intolerance*, eds. Brostoff, J. and Challacombe, S.J. (eds.) Baillière Tindall, Eastbourne. {RV}{BB}

61. Haavik, S. *et al.* (1979) Effects of the Feingold diet on seizures and hyperactivity: a single subject analysis. *J Behav Med*, 2(4): 365–74. {CN}

62. Converse, M.L., Converse, T.A. and Dall, L.D. (1991) Cervicocranial adjustments in seizure management: a case report. *Dig Chirop Econ*, 33(4): 27–8. {CN}

63. Goodman, R.J. and Mosby, J.S. (1990) Cessation of a seizure disorder: correction of the atlas subluxation complex. *Chiropractic*, 6(2): 43–6. {CN}

64. Harvey, R.F., Gunary, R.M., Hinton, R.A. and Barry, R.C. (1989) Individual and group hypnotherapy in treatment of refractory irritable bowel syndrome. *Lancet*, i(8635): 424–5. {TR}

65. Whorwell, P.J., Prior, A. and Faragher, E.B. (1984) Controlled trial of hypnotherapy in the treatment of severe refractory irritable bowel syndrome. *Lancet*, ii(8414): 1232. {TR}

66. Whorwell, P.J., Prior, A. and Colgan, S.M. (1987) Hypnotherapy in severe irritable bowel syndrome: a further experience. *Gut*, 28(4): 423–5. {TR}

67. Somper, J.D. (1988) Some cases involving the use of bowel nosodes. *Br Hom J* 77(2): 82–90. {CN}

68. Zwetchkenbaum, J. and Burakoff, R. /1988) The irritable bowel syndrome and food hypersensitivity. *Ann Allergy*, 61(1): 47–9. {TR}

69. Alun-Jones, V.A. *et al.* (1982) Food intolerance: a major factor in the pathogenesis of irritable bowel syndrome. *Lancet*, ii: 1115–7. {TR}

70. Dew, M.J. *et al.* (1984) Peppermint oil and irritable bowel syndrome. *Br J Clin Pract*, 38; 394–8. {TR}

71. Null, G. (1988) Hyperactivity and learning disabilities. *J Chiropractic*, 25(23): 34–8. {CN}
72. Spreiser, P.T. (1987) Learning disabilities – Part II. *Dig Chirop Econ*, 31(3): 20–5. {CN}
73. McPhail, C.H. and Chamove, A.S. (1989) Relaxation reduces disruption in mentally handicapped adults. *J Ment Defic Res*, 33(5): 399–406. {TR}
74. Lindsay, W.R. and Baty, F.J. (1989) Group relaxation training with adults who are mentally handicapped. *Behav Psychother*, 17(1): 43–51. {CN}
75. Lindsay, W.R., Richardson, I. and Michie, A.M. (1989) Short-term generalised effects of relaxation training on adults with moderate and severe mental handicaps. *Ment Handicap Res*, 2(6): 197–206. {TR}
76. Pruess, J.B. (1989) Vitamin therapy and children with Down's Syndrome. *Except Child*, 55(4): 336–49. {RV}
77. Uma, K. *et al* (1989) The integrated approach of yoga; a therapeutic tool for mentally retarded children: a one year controlled study. *J Ment Defic Res*, 33(5): 415–21. {TR}
78. Hubbard, E.W. (1965) Results with the potentized simillium in retarded children. *J Am Inst Hom*, 58(11–12): 338–42. {CN}
79. Griggs, W.B. (1968) Normalizing abnormal children. *J Am Inst Hom*, 61(10–12): 235–8. {CN}
80. Swayne, J. (1989) The homoeopathic treatment of behaviour disorders in adults with mental handicap. *Homoeopathy*, 39(2): 35–9. {CN}
81. Negley-Parker, E. and Araoz, D.L. (1986) Hypnotherapy with families of chronically ill children. *Int J Psychosom*, 33(2): 9–11. {CN}
82. Payne, M.B. (1989) The use of therapeutic touch with rehabilitation clients. *Rehabil Nurs*, 14(2): 69–72. {CN}
83. Lawrence, D.J. (ed.) (1991) *Fundamentals of Chiropractic*. Williams and Wilkins, Baltimore.
84. Monajem, R. (1989) Treatment of two cases of ALS. *Am J Acup*, 17(3): 205–8. {CN}
85. Meinck, H.M., Schonle, P.W. and Conrad, B. (1989) Effects of cannabinoids on spasticity and ataxia in multiple sclerosis. *J Neurol*, 236(2): 120–2. {CN}
86. Lansley, V. (1985) Homoeopathy and multiple sclerosis. *Homoeopathy*, 35(3–4): 48–9. {CN}

87. Saine, A. (1990) Homoeopathic treatment of the multiple sclerosis patient. *Homoeopath*, 10(1): 20–2. {CN}
88. Orthonos, A., Papconstantinoy, G. and Diomantidis, S.
(1988) Homoeopathic treatment of multiple sclerosis.
*Proceedings of the 43rd Congress of the International
Homoepathic Medical League*: 78–85. {TR}
89. Steinberger, A. (1986) Specific irritabiilty of acupuncture
points as an early symptom of multiple sclerosis. *Am J
Chin Med*, 14(3–4); 175–8. {CN}
90. Smith, M.O. and Rabinowitz, N. (1986) Acupuncture
treatment of multiple sclerosis: Two detailed clinical
presentations. *Am J Acupunct* 14(2): 143–6. {CN}
91. Swank, R.L. (1970) Multiple sclerosis: 20 years on a low
fat diet. *Arch Neurol*, 23: 460–74. {TR} {RV}
92. Dworkin, R.H. *et al.* (1984) Linoleic aid and multiple
sclerosis: a reanalysis of 3 double blind trials. *Neurology*,
34: 1441–45. {RV}
93. Mertin, H. and Meade, C.J. (1977) Relevance of fatty
acids in multiple sclerosis. *Br Med Bull*, 33: 67–71. {TR}
94. Fitzgerald, G.E. *et al.*, (1987) The effect of nutritional
counselling on dietary compliance and disease curse in
multiple sclerosis patients over three years. In: *Multiple
Sclerosis: Immunological, Diagnostic and Therapeutic Aspects*,
Clifford Row, F. (ed.) John Libbey, London. {TR}
95 Gypser, K.H. (1988) Myasthenia gravis – Natrum
muriaticum. *Br Hom J*, 77: 187. {CN}
96. Ramakrishnan, AU (1987) Diseases of the spine. *Br Hom
J*, 76: 221. {CN}
97. Pai, P.N. (1990) Parkinson's disease and homoeopathy.
Br Hom J, 79: 243. {CN}
98. Nishimoto, T., Ishikawa, T., Matsumoto, K. and Fujioka,
A. (1987) Efficacy of acupuncture treatment in autonomic
ataxia. *Am J Chin Med*, 15(3–4): 133–8. {CN}
99. Grier, A.R. and Proctor, D.J. (1988) Chiropractic management of a patient wiht arthritis associated with systemic
lupus erythematosus. *Pain Clinic*, 81(3): 113–8. {CN}
100. Taylor, M.R. (1990) Fibromyalgia syndrome: a literature
review. *Am J Chirop Med*, 3(3): 118–26. {CN}
101. Kirstein, A.E., Dietz, F. and Hwang, S.M. (1991)
Evaluating the safety and potential use of a weight
bearing exercise, tai chi chuan, for rheumatoid arth-

ritis patients. *Am J Phys Med Rehab*, 70(3): 136–141. {TR}

102. Strauus, G.D. *et al*. (1986) Group therapies for rheumatoid arthritis. *Arth Rheum*, 29(10): 1203–9. {TR}

103. Shearn, M.A. and Fireman, B.H. (1985) Stress management and mutual support groups in rheumatoid arthritis. *Am J Med*, 78(5): 771–5. {TR}

104. Jackson, T. (1991) An evaluation of the Mitchell method of simple physiological relaxation for women with rheumatoid arthritis. *Br J Occup Ther*, 54(3): 105–7. {TR}

105. Anon (1991) Yoga relieves RA. *Pulse*, May 25: 18. {TR}

106. Yousufzai, N.M. (1989) Rheumatoid arthritis and hypnosis: a case report. *Br J Exp Clin Hypn*, 6(3): 178–81. {CN}

107. Flor, H., Haag, G. and Turk, D.C. (1986) Long term efficacy of EMG feedback for chronic rheumatic back pain. *Pain*, 27(2): 64–70. {TR}

108. Beri, D., Malaviya, A.N., Shandilya, R. and Singh, R.R. (1988) Effect of dietary restrictions on disease activity in rheumatoid arthritis. *Ann Rheum Dis*, 47(1): 69–72. {TR}

109. Darlington, L.G., Ramsey, N.W. and Mansfield, J.R. (1986) Placebo controlled, blind study of dietary manipulation therapy in rheumatoid arthritis. *Lancet*, 1 (8475): 236–8. {TR}

110. van de Laar, M.A.F.J. *et al*. (1992) Food intolerance in rheumatoid arthritis. I: a double-blind, controlled trial of the clinical effects of the elimination of milk allergens and azo dyes. *Ann Rheum Dis*, 51(3): 298–302. {TR}

111. van de Laar M.A.F.J., *et al*. (1992) Food intolerance in rheumatoid arthritis II: Clinical and histological aspects. *Ann Rheum Dis*, 51(3): 303–6. {CN} {LAB}

112. Little, C.H., Stewart, A.G. and Fennessy, M.R. (1983) Platelet serotonin release in rheumatoid arthritis. *Lancet*, (8345): 297. {TR}

113. Parke, A.L. and Hughes, G.R.V. (1981) Rheumatoid arthritis and food. *Br Med J*, 282: 2027. {CN}

114. Fowler, P. (1989) Diet and rheumatoid arthritis. *Rheumatol Pract*, 7(1): 7–9. {RV}

115. Felder, M., De Blecourt, A.C. and Wuthrich, B. (1987) Food allergy in patients with rheumatoid arthritis. *Clin Rheumatol*, 6(2): 181–4. {TR}

116. Darlington, L.G. (1985) Does food intolerance have any role in the aetiology and management of rheumatoid disease? *Ann Rheum Dis*, 44(11): 801–4. {RV}

117. Jewett, D.L., Fein, G. and Greenberg, M.H. (1990) A double blind study of symptom provocation to determine food sensitivity. *New Eng J Med*, 323: 429–33. {TR}

118. Panusch, R.S. (1990) Food induced arthritis: clinical and serological studies. *J Rheumatol*, 17: 291–4. {TR}

119. Panusch, R.S. (1983) Diet therapy for rheumatoid arthritis. *Arth Rheum*, 26: 462–8. {TR}

120. Skjoldstom, L. (1987) Fasting and vegan diet in rheumatoid arthritis. *Scand J Rheumatol*, 15(2): 219–21. {TR}

121. Sundquist, T., Lindstrom, F. and Magnusson, K.E. (1982) Influence of fasting on intestinal permeability and disease activity in patients with rheumatoid arthritis. *Scand J Rheumatol*, 11(1): 33–8. {TR}

122. Lithell, H. *et al.* (1983) A fasting and vegetarian diet treatment trial on chronic inflammatory diseases. *Acta Derm Venereol*, 63: 397–403. {TR}

123. Uden, A.M. *et al.* (1983) Neutrophil functions and clinical performance after total fasting in patients with rheumatoid arthritis. *Ann Rheum Dis*, 42(1): 45–51. {TR}

124. Panusch, R. S. *et al.* (1986) Food-induced (allergic) arthritis. *Arth Rheum*, 29(2): 220–26. {CN}

125. Grant, M., Engelhart, K., Bray, C. and Wotjulewski, J.A. (1987) A study of dietary elimination and food challenge in rheumatoid arthritis. In *Food Allergy and Intolerance*, Brostoff, J. and Challacombe, S.J. (eds.) Bailliere Tindall, Eastbourne. {TR}

126. Hicklin, J.A. *et al.*, (1980) The effect of diet in rheumatoid arthritis. *Clin. Allergy*, 10: 463. {TR}

127. Skoldstam, L. *et al.* (1979) Effects of fasting and lacto-vegetarian diet on rheumatoid arthritis. *Scand J Rheumatol*, 8: 249–55. {TR}

128. Cooke, H.M. and Reading, C.M. (1985) Dietary intervention in SLE. *Int Clin Nutr Rev*, 5(4): 166–76. {CN}

129. Rea, W.J. and Brown, O.D. (1985) Mechanisms of environmental vascular triggering. *Clin Ecology*, 3(3): 122–8. {CN}

130. Bradley, L.A. *et al.* (1987) Effects of psychological therapy on pain behaviour of rheumatoid arthritis patients:

treatment outcome and 6 month follow up. *Arth Rheum*, 30(10): 1105–14. {TR}

131. Mandell, M. and Comte, A.A. (1982) The role of allergy in arthritis, rheumatism and polysymptomatic cerebral, visceral and somatic disorders: a double blind study. *J. Int Acad Prev Med*, (11): 5–16. {TR}

132. Werbach, M.R. (1988) *Nutritional Influences on Health*. Thorson, Wellingborough. {RV} {M} {BB}

133. Darlington, L.G. and Ramsey, N.W. (1991) Diets for rheumatoid arthritis (letter). *Lancet*, 338: 1209. {CN}

134. Helliewell, P.S. and Aremilak, T.T. (1991) Diets for rheumatoid arthritis (letter). *Lancet*, 338: 1209–10. {CN}

135. Delamere, J.P. *et al.* (1983) Jejuno-ileal bypass anthropathy: its clinical features and associations. *Ann Rheum Dis*, 42: 553–7. {CN}

136. Lucas, C. and Power, L. (1981) Dietary fat aggravates active rheumatoid arthritis. *Clin Res*, 29(4): 754A {TR}

137. Brszeski, M., Madhok, R. and Capell, H.A. (1991) Evening primrose oil in patients with rheumatoid arthritis and side-effects of non-steroidal anti-inflammatory drugs. *Br J Rheumatol*, 30(5): 370–2. {TR}

138. Cleland, L.G., French, J.K., Betts, W.H., Murphy, G.A. and Elliot, M.U. (1988) Clinical and biochemical effects of dietary fish oil supplements in rheumatoid arthritis. *J Rheumatol*, 15: 1471–5. {TR}

139. Panusch, R.S. (1987) Nutritional therapy for rheumatic diseases. *Ann Intern Med*, 106(4): 619–21. {RV}

140. Belch, J.J., Ansell, D., Madhok, R., O'Dowd, A. and Sturrock, R.D. (1988) Effects of altering dietary essential fatty acids on requirements for non-steroidal anti-inflammatory drugs in patients with rheumatoid arthritis: a double blind placebo controlled trial. *Ann Rheum Dis*, 47(2): 96–104. {TR}

141. Jantti, J., Nikkari, T., Solakivi, T., Vapaatalo, H. and Isomarki, H. (1989) Evening primrose oil in rheumatoid arthritis: changes in serum lipids and fatty acids. *Ann Rheum Dis*, 48(2): 124–7. {TR}

142. Bhatt-Sanders, D. (1985) Acupuncture for rheumatoid arthritis: an analysis of the literature. *Semin Arthritis Rheum*, 14(4): 225–31. {RV}

143. Feng, S.F., Fang, L. and Bao, G.O. (1985) Treatment of

systemic lupus erythematosus by acupuncture. A preliminary report of 25 cases. *Chin Med J*, 98(3): 171–6. {TR}

144. Yusheng, C. and Xiue, H. (1985) Auriculo-acupuncture in 15 cases of discoid lupus erythematosus. *J Tradit Chin Med*, 5(4): 261–2. {CN}

145. Fengshan, Z. and Ping, S. (1985) Blood chemistry in deficiency of kidney-yin and deficiency of kidney-yang types of sub-acute systemic lupus erythematosus. *J Tradit Chin Med*, 5(4): 265–6. {CN}

146. Yongjiang, X., Yunxing, P., Guiling, C., Xiandong, X., Ligong, L. and Guanren, H. (1986) Acupuncture treatment of early rheumatoid arthritis. *J Trad Chin Med*, 6(3): 162–4. {TR}

147. Fisher, P., Greenwood, A., Huskisson, E.C., Turner, P. and Belon, P. (1989) Effect of homoeopathic treatment of fibrositis (primary fibromyalgia) *Br Med J*, 299 (6695): 365–6. {TR}

148. Shipley, M., Berry, H., Broster, G. *et al.* (1983) Controlled trial of homoeopathic treatment of osteoarthritis. *Lancet*, i: 97–8. {TR}

149. King, S. (1988) The homoeopathic treatment of patients receiving ongoing prednisone therapy. *J Am Inst Hom*, 81(3): 113–8. {CN}

150. Audrale, L.E.C., Attra, E., da Silva, M.S.M. and Castro, A. (1988) *Randomised double blind trial with homoeopathy and placebo on rheumatoid arthritis.* Sao Paulo, Brazil: Escola Paulista da Medicine. {TR}

151. Gibson, S. (1987) A combined approach to arthritis. *Br Hom J*, 76(4); 224–6 {CN}

152. Gibson, R.G., Gibson, S.L., MacNeill, A.D. and Watson Buchanan, W. (1980) Homoeopathic therapy in rheumatoid arthritis: Evaluation by double blind clinical therapeutic trial. *Br J Clin Pharmacol*, 9: 453–9. {TR}

153. Jack, R.A. (1991) Seven successful clinical cases. *Br Hom J*, 80(2): 101–7. {CN}

154. Fisher, P. (1990) Research into homoeopathic treatment of rheumatological disease: why and how? *Complement Med Res*, 4(3): 34–40. {RV}

155. Morton, G. (1982) Arthritis and rheumatism. *Br Hom J*, 71: 105. {CN}

156. Bai, H. (1989) The short term effect on childhood rheumatoid arthritis treated with combined with western and Chinese herbal drugs. *J Tradit Chin Med*, 9(2): 108–110. {TR}

157. Zhoa, X. and Ding, J. (1988) Kidney invigorating medicine in the treatment of osteoarthritis: an experimental study. *J. Tradit Chin Med*, 8(4): 285–92. {TR}

158. Tao, X.L., Sun, Y., Dong, Y., Xiao, Y.L., Hu, D.W., Shi, Y.P., Zhu, Q.L., Dai, H. and Zhang, N.Z. (1989) A prospective, controlled, double-blind, cross-over study of Tripterygium wilfodii hook F in treatment of rheumatoid arthritis. *Chin Med J*, 102(5): 327–32. {TR}

159. Kulkani, R.R., Patki, P.S., Jog, V.P., Gandage, S.G. and Patwardhan, B. (1991) Treatment of osteoarthritis with a herbomineral formulation: a double-blind, placebo-controlled, cross-over study. *J Ethnopharmacol*, 33(1–2): 91–5. {TR}

160. Kweifio-Okai, G. (1991) Anti-inflammatory activity of a Ghanaioan anti-arthritic herbal preparation: II. *J Ethnopharmacol*, 33(1–2): 129–33. {LAB}

161. Arthur, B.E., Nykoliation, J.W. and Cassidy, J.D. (1985) Adult idiopathic scoliosis. *Eur J Chirop*, 34: 46–53. {TR} {CN}

162. Betge, G. (1985) Scoliosis correction. *Eur J Chirop*, 33: 71–91. {CN}

163. Lysaght, R. and Bodenhammer, E. (1990) Use of relaxation training to enhance functional outcomes in adults with traumatic head injuries. *Am J Occup Ther*, 44(9): 797–802. {CN}

164. Bodenhamer, E., Colename, C. and Achterberg, J. (1986) Self-directed EMG training for the control of pain and spasticity in paraplegia: a case study. *Biofeedback Self-Regul*, 11(3): 199–205. {CN}

165. Dunn, M., Davis, J. and Webster, J. (1980) Muscle spasticity: voluntary control with EMG biofeedback in quadriplegic patients. *Am J Clin Biofeedback*, 3: 5–10. {CN}

166. Rose, M., Robinson, J.E., Ells, P. and Cole, J.D. (1991) Pain following spinal cord injury: results from a postal survey. *J Tissue Viability*, 1(4): 95–8. {CN}

167. Ginsburg, C. (1986) The Shake-A-Leg body awareness training program: Dealing with spinal injury and recovery in a new setting. *Somatics*, 5(4): 31–42. {CN}

168. Du, X. (1990) Clinical observation on acupuncture treatment of 200 cases of hemiplegia. *Int J Clin Acup*, 1(3): 229–33. {TR}

169. Zhang, B. (1987) Therapeutic effects of point-through-point acupuncture in 70 cases of apoplectic hemiplegia. *J Tradit Chin Med*, 7(3): 167-8. {CN}

170. Zhang, W., Li, S., Chen, G., Zhang, Q. and Wang, Y. (1987) Acupuncture treatment of apoplectic hemiplegia. *J Tradit Chin Med*, 7(3): 157-60. {TR}

171. Shentian, S., Shurong, L. and Yongzhi, Z. (1985) Clinical study on 550 cases of cerebro-vascular hemiplegia treated by acupuncture through baihui to qubin. *J Tradit Chin Med*, 5(3): 167-70. {TR}

172. Zhang, Z. (1989) Efficacy of acupuncture in the treatment of post-stroke aphasia. *J Tradit Chin Med*, 9(2): 87-9. {TR}

173. Chen, Y.M. and Fang, Y.A. (1990) 108 cases of hemiplegia caused by stroke: the relationship between CT scan results, clinical findings and the effect of acupuncture treatment. *Acupunct Electrotherap Res*, 15(1): 9-17. {TR}

174. Ding, Y. and He, X. (1986) Traditional Chinese herbs in the treatment of neurological and neurosurgical disorders. *Can J Neurol Sci*, 13(3): 210-13. {CN}

175. Holroyd, J. and Hill, A. (1989) Pushing the limits of recovery: hypnotherapy with a stroke patient. *Int J Clin Exp Hypn*, 37(2): 120-8. {CN}

176. Margianiello, A.J. (1986) Hypnotherapy in the rehabilitation of a stroke victim: a case study. *Am J Clin Hypn*, 29(1): 64-8. {CN}

177. Sun, D., Jiang, J., Wang, D., Diao, J., Yang, X., Cheng, Y. and Zhang, T. (1987) Effects of traditional Chinese medicine of different treatment principles on hemagglutination and adhesion of uropathogenic *Escherichia coli* to uroepithelial cells. *J Tradit Chin Med*, 7(1): 53-6. {LAB}

178. Chang, P. (1988) Urodynamic studies in acupuncture for women with frequency, urgency and dysuria. *J Urol*, 140(3): 563-6. {TR}

179. Ellis, N., Briggs, R. and Dowson, D. (1990) The effect of acupuncture on noctural urinary frequency and incontinence in the elderly. *Complement Med Res*, 4(1): 16-7. {TR}

180. Buchmann, W., (1989) Diseases of the kidneys and urinary tract. *Br Hom J*, 78: 51. {CN}

181. Dickerson, C.R. (1987) Cervical manipulation: how much of a risk for stroke? *J Chiropractic*, 24(8): 63–9. {CN}
182. Peacher, W.G. (1975) Adverse reactions, contraindications and complications of acupuncture and moxibustion. *Amer J Chin Med*, 3(1): 35–46. {CN}
183. Chitgau, R. (1975) Beth Ann and Macrobioticism. In *The New Journalism*, Wolfe, T. and Johnson, E.W. (eds.) Pan, London.
184. BMA (1986) Appendix A in the British Medical Association's *Report on Alternative Therapy*. {RV}
185. Dvorak, J. and Orelli, F. (1985) How dangerous is manipulation to the cervical spine? *Manual Med*, 2(1): 1–4. {RV}
186. Sethi, T.J., Kemeny, D.M., Tobin, S., Lessof, M.H. Lambourn, E. and Bradley, A. (1986) How reliable are commercial allergy tests? *Lancet*, 1(8523): 92–4. {TR}
187. Werbach, M.R. (1986) *Third Line Medicine*. Arkana, London. {M} {RV}
188. White, L., Tursky, B. and Schwartz, G.E. (eds.) (1985) *Placebo: Theory, Research and Practice*. The Gulford Press, New York. {RV} {M}
189. Reilly, D.T., Taylor, M.A., McSharry, C. and Aitchison, T. (1986) Is homoeopathy a placebo response? Controlled trial of homocopathic potency, with pollen in hay fever as a model. *Lancet*, ii: 881–6. {TR}
190. Ferley, J.P., Zmitrou, D., D'Admehar, and Balducci, F. (1989) A controlled evaluation of a homoeopathic preparation in the treatment of influenza-like syndromes. *Br J Clin Pharmacol*, 27: 329–35. {TR}
191. Kleijnen, J., Knipschild, P. and ter Riet, G. (1991) Clinical trials of homoeopathy. *Br Med J*, 302: 316–23. {RV} {BB}
192. Koes, B.W., Assendelft, W.J., van der Heijen, G.J.M.B., Bouter, L.M. and Knipschild, P.G. (1991) Spinal manipulation and mobilisation for back and neck pain: a blinded review. *Br Med J*, 303: 1298–303. {RV} {BB}
193. Knipschild, P. (1988) Looking for gall bladder disease in the patient's iris. *Br Med J*, 297: 1578. {TR}
194. Gowania, H.J. *et al.* (1987) The effect of chamomile on wound healing – a controlled clinical-experimental double-blind trial. *Z Hautkr*, 62 (17): 1262–71. {TR}
195. Moran, A. *et al.* (1989) Analgesic, anti-pyretic and anti-

inflammatory activity of the essential oil of *Artemisia caerulescens subsp. gallicia. J Ethnopharmacol*, 27(3): 307–17.

196. Blackwell, A.L. (1991) Tea tree oil and anaerobic (bacterial) vaginosis (letter). *Lancet*, 337(8736): 300. {CN}

197. Leathwood, Chauffaud, F. (1985) Aqueous extract of valerian reduces latency to fall asleep in man. *Planta Medica*, 144–8. {TR}

198. Shehan, M.P. and Atherton, D.J. (1992) A controlled trial of traditional Chinese medicinal plants in widespread non-exudative eczema. *Br J Dermatol*, 126(2): 179–84. {TR}

199. Grayson, M.F. (1986) Manipulation in back disorders. *Br Med J (Clin Res)*, 293(6560): 1481–2. {RV} {BB}

200. Gibson, T. *et al.* (1985) Controlled comparison of short-wave diathermy in non-specific low back pain. *Lancet*, 1(8440): 1258–61. {TR}

201. Meade, T.W., Dyer, S., Browne, W., Townsend, J. and Frank, A. (1990) Low back pain of mechanical origin: randomised comparison of chiropractic and hospital out-patient treatment. *Br Med J*, 300: 143–7. {TR}

202. Doutremepuich, C. (ed.) (1991) *Ultra Low Doses*, Taylor & Francis, London. {M} {TR} {LAB}

203. Steven, C. (1991) *Experimental Studies in the Alexander Technique*. Centerline Press, Downey, California. {RV} {BB}{M}

204. Trojan, A. (1989) Benefits of self-help groups: a survey of 232 members from 65 disease-related groups. *Soc Sci Med*, 29(2): 225–32. {TR}

205. Benor, D.J. (1990) Survey of spiritual healing research. *Complement Med Res*, 4(3): 9–33. {RV} {BB}

206. Glik, D.C. (1986) Psychosocial wellness amongst spiritual healing participants. *Soc Sci Med*, 22(5); 579–86. {TR}

207. Beutler, J.J. *et al.* (1988) Paranormal healing and hypertension. *Br Med J*, 296: 1491–4. {TR}

208. Kramer, N.A. (1990) Comparison of therapeutic touch and casual touch in stress reduction of hospitalised children. *Paediatr Nurs*, 16(5): 483–5. {TR}

209. Keller, E. and Bzdek, V.M. (1986) Effects of therapeutic touch on tension headache pain. *Nurs Res*, 35(2): 101–6. {TR}

210. Swanson, B., Cronin-Stubbs, D. and Sheldon, J.A. (1989) The Impact of psychosocial factors on adapting to

physical disability: a review of the research literature. *Rehab Nursing*, 14(2): 64–8. {RV} {BB}

211. Segal, J. (1991) Why offer counselling? In *Multiple Sclerosis: Approaches to Management*. De Souza, L. (ed.) Chapman & Hall, London. {CN}

212. Paulley, J.W. (1976) Psychological management of multiple sclerosis. *Psychother Psychosom*, 27: 26–40. {CN}

213. Crawford, J.D. and McIvor, G.D. (1985) Group psychotherapy: benefits in multiple sclerosis. *Arch Phys Med Rehab*, 66: 810–13. {TR}

214. Hyman, M.D. (1975) Social and psychological factors affecting disability among ambulatory patients. *J Chron Dis*, 28: 199–216. {TR}

215. Maas, A.G. and Hogenhuis, L.A. (1987) Multiple sclerosis and possible relationship with cocoa: a hypothesis. *Ann Allergy*, 59(1): 76–9. {CN}

216. Wilson, H. *et al.* (1982) Personality characteristics and multiple sclerosis. *Psychological Reports*, 51: 791–806. {TR}

217. Grant, I. *et al.* (1989) Severely threatening events and married life difficulties preceding onset or exacerbation of multiple sclerosis. *J Neurol Neurosurg Psychiat*, 52: 8–13. {TR}

218. Hamsden, E.L. and Taylor, L.J. (1988) Stress and anxiety in the disabled patient. *Phys Ther*, 68(6): 992–6. {CN}

219. Turner R.J. and Beiser, M. (1990) Major depression and depressive symptomatology among the physically disabled: assessing the role of chronic stress. *J Nerv Mental Dis*, 178(6): 343–50. {TR}

220. Zeldow, P.B. *et al.* (1984) Physical disability, life stress and psychological adjustment in multiple sclerosis. *J Nerv Ment Dis*, 172(2): 80–4. {CN}

221. Evans, R.L. *et al.* (1985) Cognitive therapy to achieve personal goals: results of telephone counselling with disabled adults. *Arch Phys Med Rehabil*, 66(10): 693–9. {TR}

222. Ivey, A.E., Bradford Ivey, M and Sinek-Doring, L. (1987) *Counselling and Psychotherapy*. Prentice Hall, New Jersey. {M} {RV}

223. Maes, S., Vingerhoets, A. and van Heck, G. (1987) The study of stress and disease. *Soc Sci Med*, 25(6): 567–78. {RV} {BB}

302   *Bibliography*

224. Ornish, D. *et al*. (1990) The lifestyle heart trial. *Lancet*, 336: 129–33. {TR}
225. Anand, B.K., China, G.S. and Singh, B. (1961) Some aspects of electroencephalographic studies in yogis. *Electroencephalography Clin Neurophysiol*, 13: 452–6. {LAB}
226. Johnston, D.W. *et al*. (1993) Effect of stress management on blood pressure in mild primary hypertension. *Br Med J*, 306: 963–6. {TR}
227. Monro, R., Ghosh, A.K. and Kalish, D. (1989) *Yoga Research Bibliography*. Yoga Biomedical Trust, Cambridge. {BB}
228. Benson, H. *et al*. (1974) Decreased blood pressure in hypertensive subjects who regularly elicited the relaxation response. *Lancet*, i: 289–91. {TR}
229. Benson, H. (1988) *The Relaxation Response*. Collins, London. {M} {RV} {BB}
230. Patel, C.H. (1975) 12 month follow up of yoga and biofeedback in the management of hypertension. *Lancet*, 1: 62–4. {TR}
231. Kirkpatrick, R.A. (1981) Witchcraft and Lupus Erythematosus. *J Am Med Assoc*, 245: 1937–8. {CN}
232. Pruitt, R.D. (1974) Death as an expression of functional disease. *Mayo Clin Pract*, 49: 627–35. {CN}
233. Van Nguyen, T. (1991) Mind, brain and immunity: a critical review. *Holistic Nurs Pract*, 5(4): 1–9. {RV}
234. Cassileth, B.R. *et al*. (1985) Psychosocial correlates of survival in advanced malignant disease. *New Eng J Med*, 312(24): 1551–5. {TR}
235. Angell, M. (1985) Disease as a reflection of the psyche. *New Eng J Med*, 312(24): 1570–2. {CN}
236. Pettingale, K.W., Morriss, T., Greer, S. and Haybittle, J.L. (1985) Mental attitudes to cancer: an additional prognostic factor. *Lancet*, i(8431): 750. {TR}
237. Kiecolt-Glaser, J.K., Glaser, R. *et al*. (1986) Modulation of cellular immunity in medical students. *J Behav Med*, 9(1): 5–21. {TR} {BB}
238. Ader, R. and Cohen, N. (1975) Behaviorally conditioned immunosuppression. *Psychosomatic Med*, 37: 333–40. {TR}
239. Speigel, D. *et al*. (1989) Effect of psychosocial treatment

on survival of patients with metastatic breast cancer. *Lancet*, ii: 888–9.

240. Solomon, G.F. *et al.* (1987) An intensive psycho-immunologic study of long surviving persons with AIDS. *Ann New York Acad Sci*, 496: 647–55. {TR}

241. Abrahamson, L.Y. (1978) Learned helplessness in humans. *J Abnorm Psych*, 87(1); 49–74. {CN}

242. Goodwin, J.S. *et al.* (1987) The effect of marital status on stage, treatment and survival of cancer patients. *J Am Med Assoc*, 258(21): 3125–30. {TR}

243. Valliant, G.E. (1979) Natural history of male psychologic health: effects of mental health on physiologic health. *New Eng J Med*, 301(23): 1249–54. {TR}

244. Janssen, A.M. *et al.* (1987) Antimicrobial activity of essential oils: 1976–1986 literature review. *Planta Med*, 53(5): 395–8. {RV}

245. Ferley, J.P., Poutigat, N., Zmirou, D., Azzopardi, Y. and Balducci, F. (1989) Prophylactic aromatherapy for supervening infections in patients with chronic bronchitis. *Phytother Res*, 3(3): 97–100.

246. Bety, B. and Thomas, O.B. (1979) Individual temperament as a predictor of health or premature disease. *John Hopkins Med J*, 144: 81–9. {TR}

247. Berkman, L.F. and Syme, S.I.. (1979) Social networks, host resistance and mortality. *Am J Epidemiol*, 109: 186–204. {TR}

248. Klerman, G.L. and Izen, J.E. (1977) The effects of grief on physical heath and general well-being. *Adv Psychosom Med*, 9: 63–104. {TR}

249. Kiecolt-Glaser, J.K. *et al.* (1985) Psychosocial enhancment of immunocompetence in a geriatric population. *Health Psychol*, 4: 25–41. {TR}

250. Grossath-Maticek, (1984) Psychotherapy research in oncology. In *Health Care and Human Behaviour*, Steptoe, A. and Matthew, A. (eds.) Academic Press, London. {TR}

251. Guggenbuhl-Craig, A. and Micklem, N. (1987) No answer to Job: reflections on the limitations of meaning in illness. In *The Meaning of Illness*, Kidel, M and Rowe-Leete, S (eds.) Routledge, London. {CN}

252. Roth, L.L. and Rosenblatt, J.S. (1965) Mammary glands

of pregnant rats: development stimulated by licking. *Science*, 151: 1043–4. {TR}

253. Solomon, G.F., Levine, S. and Kraft, J.K. (1968) Early experiences and immunity. *Nature*, 220: 821–3. {TR}

254. Levine, S. (1960) Stimulation in infancy. *Scientific American*, 202:81–6. {TR}

255. Kaada, B. and Torsteinbo, O. (1989) Increase in plasma beta-endorphins in connective tissue massage. *Gen Pharmacol*, 20(4): 487–9.{TR}

256. Dossetor, D.R., Couryer, S. and Nicol, A.R. (1991) Massage for very self-injurious behaviour in a girl with Cornelia de Lange syndrome. *Dev Med Child Neurol*, 33(7): 636–40.

257. Fuller, J.L. (1967) Experiential deprivation and later behaviour. *Science*, 158: 1645–52. {TR}

258. Harlow, H.F. and Zimmermann, R.R. (1958) The development of affectional responses in infant monkeys. *Proc Am Philos Soc*, 102: 501–9. {TR}

259. Sokoloff, N., Yaffe, S., Weintraub, D. and Blase, B. (1969) Effects of handling on the subsequent development of premature infants. *Developmental Psychol*, 1: 765–8. {TR}

260. Acolet, D. *et al.* (1993) Changes in plasma cortisol and catecholamine concentrations in response to massage in preterm neonates. *Arch Dis Child*, 68(1 suppl): 29–31. {TR}

261. Reed, B.V. and Held, J.M. (1988) Effects of sequential connective tissue massage on autonomic nervous system of middle-aged and elderly adults. *Phys Ther*, 68(8): 1231–4.

262. Bernstein, L. (1957) The effects of variation in handling upon learning and retention. *J Comparative Physiol Psychol*, 50: 162–7. {TR}

263. Temerlin, M.K. *et al.* (1967) Effects of increased mothering and skin contact on retarded boys. *Am J Mental Deficiency*, 71: 890–93. {CN}

264. Naliboff, B.D. and Tachiki, K.H. (1991) Autonomic and skeletal muscle responses to nonelectrical cutaneous stimulation. *Percept Mot Skills*, 72(2): 575–84.

265. Vormbrock, J.K. and Grossberg, J.M. (1988) Cardiovascular effects of human–pet dog interactions. *J Behav Med*, 11(5): 509–17. {TR}

266. Culliton, B.J. (1987) Take two pets and call me in the morning. *Science*, 237 (4822); 1560–61. {RV}

267. Field, T. *et al.* (1992) Massage reduces anxiety in child and adolescent psychiatric patients. *J Am Acad Child Adolesc Psychiatry*, 31(1): 125–31. {TR}
268. Field, T. *et al.* (1986) Tactile/kinesthetic stimulation effects on preterm neonates. *Paediatrics*, 77(5): 654–8. {TR}
269. Siegel, B.S. (1986) *Love, Medicine and Miracles*. Rider, London. {M}
270. Selye, H. (1978) *The Stress of Life*. McGraw-Hill, New York. {M} {BB}
271. Montagu, A. (1978) *Touching: The Human Significance of the Skin*. Harper and Row, New York. {M} {BB}
272. Sanderson, H., Harrison, J. and Price, S. (1991) *Aromatherapy and massage for people with learning difficulties*. Hands On Publishing, Birmingham. {M} {CN} {BB}
273. Hunter, J. and Lee, A. (1990) Nature's answer to irritable bowel. *Doctor*, Nov 22. 47. {TR}
274. Gay, D., Dick, G. and Upton, G. (1986) Multiple sclerosis associated with sinusitis: a case-controlled study in general practice. *Lancet*, i(8485): 851–9. {TR}
275. Garrow, J.S. (1988) Applied kinesiology and food allergy. *Br Med J*, 296: 1573. {TR}
276. Kenney, J.J., Clemens, R. and Forsythe, K.D. (1988) Applied kinesiology unreliable for assessing nutrient status. *J Am Diet Assoc*, 88: 698–704. {TR}
277. O'Farrelly, C. *et al.* (1988) Association between villous atrophy in rheumatoid arthritis and rheumatoid factor and gliadin-specific IgG. *Lancet*, ii: 819–23. {TR} {LAB}
278. Basset, I.B., Pannowitz, D.L. and Barnetson, R.S. (1990) A comparative study of tea-tree oil versus benzoyl-peroxide in the treatment of acne. *Med J Aust*, 153(8): 455–8. {TR}
279. Barel, S. *et al.* (1991) The anti-microbial activity of the essential oil from *Achillea fragantissima*. *J Ethnopharmacol*, 33(1–2): 187–91. {LAB}
280. Buchbauer, G. *et al.* (1991) Aromatherapy: evidence for sedative effects of the essential oil of lavender after inhalation. *Z Naturforsc*, 46(11–12): 1067–72. {LAB}
281. Torri, S. *et al.* (1988) Contingent negative variaton (CNV) and the psychological effects of odour. In *Perfumery: The Psychology and Biology of Fragrance*, Van Toller, S. and Dodd, G.H. (eds.) Chapman & Hall, London. {TR}

282. Wang Zhao-Pu (1991) *Acupressure Therapy*. Churchill-
      Livingstone, Edinburgh.

Index

THE LIBRARY
GUILDFORD COLLEGE
of Further and Higher Education

140134